ATIONS
OF AIDS
ILDREN
N CARE

PUBLISHED BY
BRITISH AGENCIES FOR
ADOPTION & FOSTERING
11 SOUTHWARK STREET
LONDON SE1 1RQ

ISBN 0 903534 72 X
ISSN 02620-082X
DESIGNED BY ANDREW HAIG
TYPESET BY ETHNOGRAPHICA
PRINTED AND BOUND BY ASHDOWN PRESS

DISCUSSION SERIES : 9

The implications of AIDS for children in care

edited by Daphne Batty

◆

Medical consultants:
Dr Anne Jepson
Chair, BAAF Medical Group Executive Committee
Dr Marion Miles
Representative, British Paediatric Association
BAAF Medical Group Executive Committee

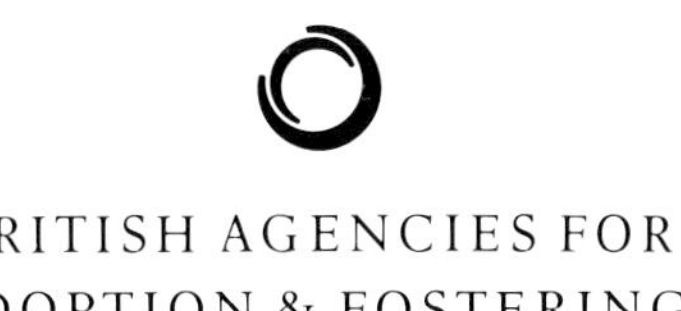

BRITISH AGENCIES FOR
ADOPTION & FOSTERING

BAAF is grateful to the Hilden Charitable Fund
for meeting the production costs of this book.

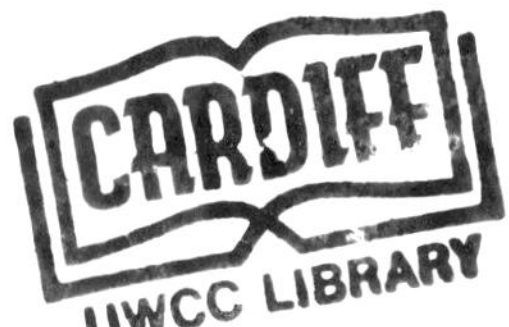

Contents

1 Introduction

Daphne Batty, Secretary to the BAAF Medical Group

About this book

Over the past 18 months BAAF has received a continuing flow of enquiries about placing children who are at risk of developing *Human Immunodeficiency Viral disease* in substitute families. In response, we invited a number of people with special experience in this field to present papers to an invited audience of representatives of various child care and medical interests, under the chairmanship of Professor John Forfar, President of the British Paediatric Association. They met in London on 14 May 1987. These papers, amended to take into account points made in the ensuing discussions, make up this publication. Information has been updated to July 1987. While it is important to remember that medical knowledge about HIV infection and AIDS is increasing rapidly (and BAAF will make every effort to keep abreast of relevant knowledge), many of the issues of principle that are considered remain constant.

In the first paper, Professor Catherine Peckham and Dr Yvonne Senturia outline the various ways the disease can be spread and the implications for the care of children. Dr Jacqueline Mok then describes the setting up and work of the Edinburgh research project which provides continuing paediatric surveillance of children born to infected mothers. She also discusses medical factors relevant to the family placement of children in care. This is followed by two papers written by members of Lothian Regional Council Social Work Department in which Anne Black sets out the issues that must be considered by child care agency management teams and Kate Skinner describes the experience of her department in preparing and supporting substitute parents caring for children at risk of HIV infection. Richard White then constructs a legal framework in the context of English law – to some extent hypothetical at this stage – within which decisions regarding children will be made.

While concern in the UK has centred mainly on young children at risk, agencies are also responsible for the welfare of older children and young people, many of whom are already sexually active. Colin Griffiths introduces this issue by discussing the education of young people about AIDS, and describes the changes that have taken place in this field over the few years since AIDS was first diagnosed in the UK in 1983. We recognise that this paper represents the tip of yet another iceberg and that BAAF, with other child care agencies, must return to this subject in the near future. Lastly we highlight some of the lessons learned at the BAAF seminar and list the issues to which agencies must address themselves in planning for children at risk of HIV infection.

As a preliminary to the more specialist contributions outlined above, this introduction attempts to summarise the main facts about AIDS. These may be familiar to some readers but it is nonetheless important to repeat them as they must now be included in the basic knowledge of practising social workers, their managers and legal advisers, as well as that of doctors concerned with families and children.

The nature of the disease

The illness is caused by the Human Immunodeficiency Virus (HIV). Two strains of the virus currently identified, HIV I and HIV II, are found in humans, and in each of these strains there are an increasing number of sub-strains. (A third main strain, STLV III, is found in African green monkeys, but links with the human strain HIV II are unclear.) HIV I is by far the most common strain in Europe and the USA, while HIV II prevails in parts of Africa.

The presence of HIV in the body leads to the suppression of certain blood cells essential for the proper functioning of the immune system (T.4 helpercells). This failure leaves the body open to the development of opportunistic infections, the most common of which in adults is *pneumocystic carinii pneumonia*, and certain tumours, most notably *Kaposi's sarcoma*. When a person suffers from one of these illnesses in the absence of any other condition causing suppression of the immune system, he or she can be diagnosed as having the *Acquired Immune Deficiency Syndrome* (AIDS).

Human beings can carry and pass on the virus without displaying any of these symptoms. They can be described as infected with HIV or, if they have been found by testing to carry antibodies to the virus, as *seropositive*. Some seropositive people may exhibit a variety of other symptoms, including herpes simplex, thrush and a persistent form of diarrhoea. The condition giving rise to these symptoms is known as the *Aids Related Complex* (ARC). ARC may exist independently of AIDS or may be a precursor to manifestations of the full syndrome.

HIV does not render the immune system powerless against all infections. The system can still operate against many of the more common viral and bacterial infections, such as influenza, as well as against more serious ones.

HIV may attack the central nervous system, causing severe brain damage, resulting in dementia and death within a year. Infection of the brain may occur separately from generalised HIV disease of the body, the individual being *seronegative.*

To sum up, the initial invasion of the body is by the Human Immunodeficiency Virus. This can lead to the condition known as the Acquired Immune Deficiency Syndrome and/or to an attack on the central nervous system, but the seropositive person's illness and possible death will be due to one of the conditions mentioned above.

Transmission of the virus

The virus has been found in significant quantities in blood, semen and vaginal secretions and in lesser quantities in saliva, breast milk and other body fluids (see Chapter 2). It is now common knowledge that the highest incidence of transmission is through penetrative sexual intercourse (although the rate of infection is uncertain) and also that the virus can be transmitted by the deliberate or accidental injection of contaminated blood or blood products, hence the high incidence of infection among intravenous drug abusers who share needles. Although the virus has been detected in saliva in the laboratory, there is at present no evidence of transmission through normal family or social contact. This statement is well documented in the paper by Professor Peckham and Dr Senturia (Chapter 2).

The percentage of seropositive people who will eventually develop the disease is still uncertain, but the 10 per cent publicised two years ago is now thought to be an underestimate. What is certain is that the virus, when outside the human body, is easy to kill. Good standards of everyday hygiene are sufficient for the care of seropositive children both at home and at school, unless either children or carers have persistent open skin lesions. Public health guidelines recommend the use of household bleach (one part to nine parts of water) for cleaning up spilled body fluids. Hot water and soap also kill this virus.

Where children are concerned, the percentage of those who are seropositive and develop the disease is also uncertain, but is likely to be higher than in adults. HIV infection can be transmitted to children through the following routes:

- infection *in utero* if the mother is seropositive
- infection during the course of the birth
- breast feeding (only one recorded case)
- transfusion of contaminated blood or blood products
- being bitten by an infected person (one recorded case*)
- sexual abuse by an infected person
- the child's own sexual activity with an infected person

Dr Mok discusses paediatric infection in some detail in Chapter 3. She also sets out (in Table 1) and discusses in her paper the spectrum of paediatric HIV disease, the initial symptoms of which are often non-specific – that is, not exclusively relating to HIV infection but common also in other diseases. Examples of non-specific symptoms are failure to thrive, diarrhoea or unexplained fever.

Treatment of the disease

Doctors are becoming more hopeful about drug treatment, but drugs currently available are very costly and have unpleasant side effects.

Testing for serostatus

The effectiveness of tests for the existence of the virus in children is discussed fully in the first two papers. It is important to note that the test most readily available in the UK at present does not identify the virus itself but the *existence of antibodies to the virus*. It must be remembered that antibodies can take several months to develop after the introduction of the virus, and also that young children born to seropositive mothers can carry their mothers' antibodies for any period up to 15 months.

A more accurate test, for antigens in the blood, is already available for adults, but for a number of medical reasons this is not practicable in its present form for children. One reason is that more blood is required

---

*and many recorded cases of bites where the victim did not become infected (known as seroconversion).

for an accurate result than can be spared from a child's body at any one time.

Confidentiality

Much has been written and said about the very real need for people at risk of HIV infection to be counselled before submitting to an antibody test, at least while the present degree of public ignorance and prejudice pertains. Guidelines issued by the BMA state that doctors responsible for testing are not free to divulge the results of a test to anyone (including other doctors) without the consent of the person tested. Experience in Scotland, however, is that seropositive mothers have been generous in allowing information to be divulged in the interests of their children and wherever possible it is advisable, as well as more accurate, to test the mother or, in the case of sexual abuse, the perpetrator, rather than the child. While social workers must also treat information as confidential, they are statutorily bound to put first the interests of the child, and could divulge social information when this is considered to be in the child's best interests.

Conclusion

At the present time (July 1987) the majority of sufferers of HIV in the UK are homosexual and bi-sexual men, intravenous drug abusers and recipients of infected blood products. Sexual partners of these people are at risk. When a judgement has to be made about exposure of a child to infection, social information, while perhaps not precise, is likely to be of more assistance at present than a test result.

2 Transmission of HIV infection: implications for fostering and adoption

Professor Catherine Peckham and Dr Yvonne Senturia

Human Immunodeficiency Virus (HIV) has been found in peripheral blood, cell-free plasma, lymph nodes, bone marrow cells, spinal fluid, brain tissue, semen, cervical and vaginal secretions, lung tissue, saliva and tears.[1] Although bodily fluids from an HIV positive individual might theoretically pose a risk of infection, epidemiological data increasingly suggest that there are only a limited number of sources and routes for spread of the virus. These include sexual intercourse with an infected individual, exposure to infected blood or blood products through transfusion or sharing needles or other equipment that allow passage of blood from one individual to another, and transmission of infection in the perinatal period from an HIV positive mother to her infant (Table 1). The relative efficiency of transmission by each of these sources is unknown.

Table 1

Ways in which HIV infection is spread
Sexual contact
Sharing of needles for IV drug abuse
Transfusion of infected blood or blood products
Infected mother to infant perinatally

AIDS surveillance in the USA

By 20 March 1987, 2227 women with AIDS had been notified to the Centers for Disease Control (CDC) in Atlanta, Georgia. Women at high

Professor Catherine Peckham is Professor of Paediatric Epidemiology with a major interest in perinatal infections.

Dr Yvonne Senturia is a paediatrician and epidemiologist with a special interest in immunisations and infectious disease.

risk include intravenous drug abusers, prostitutes, women from countries where HIV prevalence is high and women with partners who fall into the high risk groups. This number has been increasing year by year, and is being mirrored by an increase in the number of children with AIDS.

By 20 March 1987, 462 children under the age of 13 years had been reported to the CDC as cases of AIDS (CDC unpublished data). 368 (80 per cent) were from high-risk families (166 had intravenous drug abusing mothers), 24 (5 per cent) were haemophiliacs, 57 (12 per cent) had received blood transfusions prior to becoming ill and for 13 (3 per cent) no risk had yet been identified.

It is important to appreciate, however, that due to the long incubation period, cases of AIDS represent only the tip of the iceberg, and reflect the size of the problem as it was three to five years ago.

Paediatric HIV and AIDS surveillance in the UK

There are two surveillance schemes in the UK: a laboratory scheme reporting confirmed HIV antibody laboratory tests in England, Wales and Northern Ireland and separately for Scotland, and a clinical reporting scheme for AIDS cases in the UK. By the end of May 1987, 126 children under the age of 15 in England, Wales and Northern Ireland were seropositive for HIV (Table 2), of whom 13 were known to have an HIV positive mother. A further 108 were haemophiliacs and two were recipients of blood products. Two were born to African parents whose HIV status was unknown, and for the remaining infant the transmission category was unknown.

Table 2

HIV antibody positive reports in children

England, Wales and Northern Ireland (7.11.84–29.5.87)

Age (years)	Male	Female	Unknown	Total
0 – 4	17	6	1	24
5 – 9	43	–	–	43
10 – 14	59	–	–	59
Total	119	6	1	126

Source: PHLS CDSC (unpublished)

In Scotland, by the end of April 1987, 46 children under the age of four were HIV seropositive, of whom 15 are known to have at least one intravenous drug abusing parent. An additional 16 boys between five and 15 years were seropositive.

Paediatric AIDS is reported either directly to the Communicable Disease Surveillance Centre (CDSC) or through notifications by paediatricians to the British Paediatric Surveillance Unit. By the end of May 1987, a total of 13 children with confirmed AIDS were known to CDSC; seven were children of HIV positive mothers, three were recipients of blood products (abroad), and three were haemophiliacs. All but two of the seven children of HIV positive mothers had been born abroad. The mother of one of the UK-born children had received a blood transfusion in Africa (PHLS CDSC unpublished).

Perinatal transmission of HIV

The great majority of identified HIV positive children are born in high-risk families. With current laboratory techniques, it is not possible to distinguish between intra-uterine, intrapartum and postnatal infection. Although there is clear evidence for intra-uterine transmission, there is only one case report where breast feeding seemed to be the most likely route of transmission.[2]

It is difficult to make a definitive diagnosis of HIV infection in an infant born to a mother known to be seropositive. This is because viral isolation is difficult and, as maternal antibody persists in the child for a considerable length of time, the presence of HIV antibody in the infant does not necessarily imply infection. Definitive categorisation of infants as infected must be delayed therefore until the second year of life, in the absence of virus isolation or *antigenaemia* at an earlier date.

Currently the natural history of perinatal HIV infection is unknown. Prospective follow-up of infants born to HIV positive mothers is required to describe the long-term sequelae of infection acquired *in utero*. Such studies are currently in progress in the USA and Europe. The European collaborative study includes children from Edinburgh, Padua and Berlin, areas where the prevalance of HIV infection among drug addicts is high.[3]

Transmission of HIV from blood products

Because of pooling of plasma from numerous blood donors for the production of clotting factor concentrates, individuals with severe haemophilia may be exposed to as many as 100,000 blood donors per year. The first case of AIDS in a haemophiliac was diagnosed in 1982. Since 1984 the risk of transmission has been markedly reduced by virus inactivation steps in the production of clotting factors, screening of donor units for HIV antibody and voluntary exclusion of high-risk groups from the donor pool. However, a large proportion of haemophiliacs in the UK are already HIV antibody positive (Table 3).[4]

Table 3

Antibody to HIV in children with haemophilia

Age (years)	Total number tested	Number (%) HIV positive
< 5	60	11 (18%)
5 – 9	149	39 (26%)
10 – 14	174	92 (53%)
15 – 19	243	125 (51%)

Adapted from UK Haemophilia Centre Directors, June 1986 British Medical Journal, Vol 293, pages 175–176.

A prospective study in France from October 1983 to November 1985 showed that an increasing proportion of severely haemophiliac children attending a boarding school were HIV positive (Table 4).[5]

Table 4

Antibody status in severe haemophiliac children in a French boarding school

Year	Total number tested	Number (%) HIV positive
1982	22	2 (9%)
1983	18	6 (33%)
1984	25	11 (44%)
1985	44	22 (50%)

Among the 15 less severe haemophiliacs, only 3 (20 per cent) were antibody positive. Although no child had developed AIDS symptoms,

immunological testing of HIV positive and HIV negative haemophiliacs and control subjects showed mild impairment of immune function in those haemophiliacs who were antibody positive.

Prospective studies are required to determine the risk of AIDS and its natural history following neonatal transfusion of blood and blood products. Amman *et al* described a 12-month male infant with AIDS who had received multiple blood products for rhesus incompatability during the first two weeks of life.[6] One of the donors, who had appeared healthy at the time of blood donation, died of AIDS 17 months later. This child was not from a high-risk family and there were no other known sources of infection. It is possible that the relative immunosuppression of the neonate could increase the risk of AIDS or hasten the progression of HIV infection.

Transmission to contacts of HIV positive individuals

Forty-two family members of 29 HIV seropositive adults and children with haemophilia were examined for HIV antibody status.[7] All family members were seronegative even though they had been exposed for an average interval of 20 months. The spouse of a seropositive adult and 23 parents of 27 seropositive children assisted regularly with home transfusions, yet no seroconversions occurred. These results suggest that the likelihood of transmission of infection from haemophiliacs is extremely low. This is consistent with the findings in the French boarding school study where none of 70 children living in close contact with haemophiliacs developed HIV antibodies.[5] Although cases of HIV infection in wives of haemophiliac men have been reported, the only children of haemophiliac men who have developed AIDS are those with mothers who are also HIV positive.

Serological studies have suggested that needle stick injuries are rarely associated with seroconversion to HIV. Longitudinal studies of accidental innoculation by health care workers in the USA have shown only one seroconversion (with minimum six month follow-up) out of 520 well-documented percutaneous or mucous-membrane exposures to blood or body fluids from patients with HIV infection.[8,9] In two of a further 369 incidents where baseline blood specimens were not available, accidentally-exposed health care workers were reported to be HIV seropositive. This combined information suggests the risk is infinitesimal. A low risk of occupational infection was also reported by a smaller prospective study in the UK where there was no evidence of transmission among 150 health care workers who had been accidentally exposed to HIV infection.[10]

In a well-designed study 101 household contacts of 39 patients diagnosed with AIDS or AIDS-Related Complex (ARC) and oral thrush were interviewed and tested.[11] The only contact who became infected was a five-year-old girl whose mother had AIDS. It is likely that the child's infection had been acquired perinatally since she had experienced symptoms compatible with HIV infection since infancy. These household contacts had substantial exposure to patients with AIDS yet none seroconverted despite the fact that they were poor, lived in overcrowded conditions and many shared household facilities. This would again indicate that the risk of horizontal transmission was minimal.

Kaplan *et al*, as part of a study of families of children with AIDS, reported that seropositive contacts were all from high-risk groups and that there were no seroconversions among adults with no risk factors for AIDS.[12] Specifically, three foster mothers and one grandmother, who had cared for seropositive children since infancy, were seronegative.

Of the over 17,000 AIDS cases reported to the Centers for Disease Control, except for sexual partners and children born to infected mothers, none of the family members are known to have contracted AIDS.[13]

The implications of HIV infection on schooling

The mode of transmission and groups at high risk of HIV infection are similar to those for hepatitis B. However, casual transmission from person to person, absent in HIV, has been reported with hepatitis B. This, together with other evidence, suggests that guidelines aimed at the control and management of hepatitis B in schools, day-care centres, hospitals, and among community workers and family contacts should be more than adequate to deal with the presence of HIV seropositive individuals in the population. We would stress that transmission of infection seems to require intimate sexual contact or the injection of infected blood products.

There have been no reports of transmission of HIV acquired by children in day-care or foster-care settings or schools.[14] Doctors looking after children at high risk, such as infants born to IV drug abusers, would be advised to make efforts to obtain parental consent for HIV testing. Known seropositive children who are incontinent, or who have severe behavioural disturbances with abnormal mouthing, chewing or biting behaviour are advised to be withheld from communal care settings due to the theoretical (but undocumented) risk of HIV transmission via bodily fluids.[15,16] The decision about whether an HIV seropositive child can attend day care should be made on an individual basis. We would not recommend widespread screening of children as a condition of entry to day nurseries or schools. This would not provide additional protection to the other children above that available from maintaining the standards of hygiene required for the control of hepatitis B in the school situation. School personnel should be trained in uniform procedures for handling blood and bodily secretions in schools to minimise transmission of HIV, hepatitis B, and other infectious agents.[16]

Evidence against the casual spread of the virus is mounting. Voluntary consent of parent or guardian is necessary for testing and confidentiality must be maintained.[17] There is no justification for breaching confidentiality by indiscriminately releasing information about HIV status to school personnel. This would only result in stigmatising the child and his or her family without benefiting classmates or staff. The only documented risk relating to HIV infection in the school setting is the personal risk, in the unusual situation of a symptomatic immunosuppressed child, of exposure to epidemic infections (such as chicken-pox or measles) within the school.[16] Ongoing epidemiological studies will serve as the basis for refining these recommendations over time.

Immunisation and HIV infection

Although live vaccines (oral polio, measles and BCG) should be withheld from children with HIV symptoms (AIDS/ARC) because of the possibility that their immune system may not be functioning properly, children without HIV symptoms should be immunised in the routine way. The importance of protecting these infants from natural disease led the World Health Organisation and the Immunisation Practices Advisory Committee of the US Public Health Service to recommend that DTP, live oral polio, and measles vaccines should be given to asymptomatic HIV seropositive children.[18,19] However, children living in a household where someone has AIDS/ARC should be given inactivated polio vaccine instead of oral polio vaccine, in order to avoid any risk of secondary transmission.

Conclusions

At the present time, there appears to be no justification for routine screening of all children prior to fostering or adoption. The screening of infants born to mothers at high risk, before adoption or foster care placement, raises unique problems. The rationale for HIV testing prior to adoption is to give potential parents the information required to make decisions about the child's medical care and to consider the possible social and psychological effects on their families.[15,20] However, antibody testing in the first year of life will not conclusively determine whether a child is infected. Moreover, a seropositive child, who may not be infected, will be difficult to place, and an infant who is seronegative may indeed be infected.

There is an inherent conflict between the stigmatisation of these at-risk children and the interests of adoptive parents who are faced with three major areas of concern:

- the potential medical complications should AIDS develop
- the stigmatisation of the family who have an HIV positive child
- the unfounded fear of transmission of infection to their family members

Further studies are required to clarify these issues and it is hoped that the rapid advances being made in virological techniques will make it possible to establish sooner whether the infant born to a high-risk mother is infected with HIV.

References

1 Peterman T A and Curran J W 'Sexual transmission of human immunodeficiency virus' *J Am Medical Assoc* 1986; 256 (16): 2222-2226.

2 Peckham C S, Senturia Y D and Ades A E 'Obstetric and perinatal consequences of human immunodeficiency virus (HIV) infection: a review' *Brit J Obstet Gynecol* 1987; 94: 403-407.

3 Mok J Q, Giaquinto C, De Rossi A, Grosch-Wörner I, Ades A E and Peckham C S 'Infants born to HIV seropositive mothers – preliminary findings from a multi-centre European study' *Lancet* 1987; i: 1164-1168.

4 United Kingdom Haemophilia Centre Directors 'Prevelance of antibody to HTLV-III in haemophiliacs in the United Kingdom' *British Medical Journal* 1986; 293: 175-176.

5 Berthier A, Fauchet R, Genetet N, Pommerevil M, Chamaret S, Fonlupt J, Gueguen M and Mentagnier L 'Transmissability of human immunodeficiency virus in haemophiliac and non-haemophiliac children living in a private school in France' *Lancet* 1986; ii: 598-601.

6 Amman A J, Cowan M J, Wara D W, Weintrub P, Dritz S, Goldman H and Perkins H A 'Acquired immunodeficiency in an infant: possible transmission by means of blood products' *Lancet* 1983; i: 956-958.

7 Lawrence D N and Mason J M 'HTLV-III/LAV Antibody status of spouses and household contacts assisting in home infusion of hemophilia patients' *Blood* 1985; 66 (3): 703-705.

8 Henderson D K, Saah A J, Zak B J, Kaslow R A, Lane C, Falks T, Blackwelder W C, Schmitt J, LaCamera D J, Masur H and Fauci A S 'Risk of nosocomial infection with human t-cell lymphotropic virus in a large cohort of intensively exposed health care workers' *Ann Intern Med* 1986; 104: 644-647.

9 McCray E 'Occupational risk of the acquired immunodeficiency syndrome among health care workers' *New Engl J Med* 1986; 314 (17): 1127-1132.

10 McEvoy M, Porter K, Mortimer P, Simmons N and Shanson D 'Prospective study of clinical, laboratory and ancillary staff with accidental exposures to blood or body fluids from patients infected with HIV' *British Medical Journal* 1987; 294: 1595-1597.

11 Friedland G H, Saltzman B R, Rogers M F, Kahl P A, Lesser M L, Mayers M M and Klein R S 'Lack of transmission of HTLV-III/LAV infection to household contacts of patients with AIDS or AIDS-related complex with oral candidiasis' *New Engl J Med* 1986; 314 (6): 344-349.

12 Kaplan J E, Oleske J M, Getchell J P, Kalyanaram V S, Minnefor A B, Zabala-Ablan M, Joshi V and Denny T 'Evidence against transmission of human T-lymphotropic virus/lymphadenopathy associated virus in families of children with the acquired immunodeficiency syndrome' *Pediatr Infect Dis J* 1985; 4 (5): 468-471.

13 Centers for Disease Control 'Apparent transmission of human T-lymphotrophic virus type III/lymphadenopathy-associated virus from a child to a mother providing health care' *Morbidity & Mortality Weekly Report* 1986; 35(5): 76-79.

14 MacDonald K L, Danila R N and Osterholm M T 'Infection with human T-lymphotropic virus type III/lymphadenopathy-associated virus: considerations for transmission in the child day care setting' *Rev Infect Dis* 1986; 8(4): 606-612.

15 Centers for Disease Control 'Education and foster care of children infected with human T-lymphotropic virus type III/lymphadenopathy-associated virus' *Morbidity & Mortality Weekly Report* 1985; 34 (34): 517-521.

16 Am Acad Pediatr 'School attendance of children and adolescents with human T lymphotrophic virus III/lymphadenopathy associated virus infection' *Pediatrics* 1986; 77 (3): 430-432.

17 Grossman M 'Human immunodeficiency virus infections in children: public health and policy issues' *Pediatric Infect Dis* 1987; 6 (1): 113-116.

18 Immunisation Practices Advisory Committee 'Immunisation of children infected with Human T-lymphotropic virus type III/lymphadenopathy associated virus' *Pediatr Infect Dis J* 1987; 6 (2): 209-212.

19 'Expanded programme on immunisation' Joint WHO/UNICEF statement on immunisation and AIDS *Weekly Epidemiological Record* 1987; 62: 53-54.

20 Bayer R, Levine C and Wolf S M 'HIV antibody screening – an ethical framework for evaluating proposed programs' *JAMA* 1986; 256 (13): 1768.

3 HIV seropositive babies – implications in planning for their future

Dr Jacqueline Mok

Introduction

The greatest risk of HIV infection in children is to be born to a mother who herself is infected with the virus. Current information suggests that the virus is transmitted from mother to infant during pregnancy, although some children have been infected through blood and blood products.

In the United Kingdom to date, only one per cent of patients with the Acquired Immune Deficiency Syndrome had intravenous drug abuse as a high-risk activity. The prevalence for HIV antibody amongst intravenous drug abusers (IVDAs) in England and Wales remains between 5 – 10 per cent, while 50 – 60 per cent of Scotland's IVDAs have been reported to be seropositive. In Edinburgh in particular, IVDAs appear to share needles more frequently and with more people. It was therefore not surprising that, when HIV was introduced into Edinburgh in late 1983, it spread rapidly.

Medical, nursing and laboratory staffs got together and drew up guidelines for management, including a co-ordinated paediatric follow-up of infants born to seropositive mothers. We realised at the time that very little was known about the natural history of perinatal HIV transmission so it was important, with the babies born in Edinburgh, that one person should co-ordinate the follow-up and I was asked to be responsible for this surveillance programme.

In January 1986 the Paediatric Counselling and Screening Clinic was started at the City Hospital. They had already, two months previously, started a counselling and screening clinic as an alternative testing site, so it was reasonable that I should have a paediatric input

---

Dr Jacqueline Mok is Consultant Paediatrician (Community) responsible for the surveillance of children born to seropositive mothers in Edinburgh. She is participating in a European collaborative study of the natural history of perinatal HIV infection, together with colleagues in Padua and Berlin.

into an existing clinic. Initially staff consisted of myself and a nurse counsellor, trained in paediatrics but not in developmental screening, that is, not a health visitor. Later we obtained the services of a health visitor who liaises between the maternity hospitals and myself so that I am informed, with consent, of all the deliveries of infants to HIV seropositive women. We hope that in future the health visitor can see the babies with me. Latterly, we have also had a dental hygienist to advise in the clinic, in the hope that caries can be prevented.

Because we knew from past experience that intravenous drug abusers were not very good at keeping clinic appointments, we decided to set up a mother-baby clinic. In this way, if we could get the mother to the clinic with the baby, an adult physician could also check on her. So the adult screening clinic refer to me the women who are seropositive and pregnant, and neonatal paediatricians inform me about deliveries. General practitioners also refer patients, especially toddlers, that is, young children who were born between 1983 and 1985 and who may have been infected because their mothers were subsequently found to be seropositive. The social work department refers children for different reasons, mainly to discuss whether children should be screened. Self-referrals have also been fairly common.

The clinic serves a dual purpose: monitoring for clinical developments and research. I see the babies initially at six weeks because all newborns have a six-week check, and then see them at three months and every three months thereafter. Time is spent on counselling and advice on normal infant care, on taking a history and on clinical examination. In this way I hope to pick up early signs and symptoms in these infants. Growth and development are documented and immunisations are discussed and supervised.

Attendance at the clinic has risen. Of all the infants I have now, 30 were born to mothers who are seropositive. Not all come to the clinic: I visit about 60 per cent at home. By going out to see them consistently I have not lost any of the infants to follow-up. A recent development has been an offer by one of the mothers with appropriate experience to run a group for mothers, and we are supporting her in this project.

Planning for the future of these children starts with antenatal care for the mothers. Resources for the routine surveillance as well as hospital care of the infants are discussed, together with day-care and foster-care. Finally an attempt is made, looking into the future, to identify problems as these children grow up.

The mothers

Evidence from the United States suggests that pregnancy accelerates the progression of AIDS in women.[1] However, the mothers in that study were identified because they had already given birth to a child with AIDS and they represent the severe end of the spectrum. Mothers of asymptomatic HIV infected children have not been studied. More thorough, prospective follow-up of both pregnant and non-pregnant HIV seropositive women from similar risk groups would resolve the present question of whether pregnancy does indeed increase the risk of development of full-blown AIDS.

Until more is known about the effect of pregnancy on HIV infection, and also because of the risk of virus transmission to the foetus, women who are HIV seropositive are advised against pregnancy or are offered termination of pregnancy. The chaotic lifestyle of most IVDAs means that this advice is usually not heeded, or that they present too advanced in pregnancy for termination to be considered. Despite what seemed adequate counselling to women who attended the clinic at the City Hospital, two women had unwanted pregnancies terminated while several others declined termination of pregnancy.

It therefore became clear that it was necessary to do more than just offer advice and expect women to attend local family planning clinics. With the help of the Family Planning Service in Edinburgh, the City Hospital Screening Clinic counsellors have attended family planning courses and the clinic now has supplies of contraceptives freely available. It remains to be seen whether these on-site facilities will result in a reduction of pregnancy rates amongst the women attending the clinic.

Perinatal care

The unpredictable lifestyles and low level of ante-natal care amongst pregnant HIV seropositive women led to anxieties about premature deliveries and low birth-weight babies with the attendant problems. While it was unlikely that an infant would be born with AIDS, infants born to seropositive women had to be assumed to be at high risk of infection. Fears, perceived and real, among medical and nursing staff were discussed in detail during several meetings and guidelines drawn up. It was decided that seropositive women should deliver wherever they were booked – that is, no maternity unit was to be singled out for these deliveries. In view of the large quantities of blood and amniotic fluid present, appropriate precautions during the delivery include protective impermeable clothing with goggles and gloves worn. The well infant is kept in the same room as the mother, while isolation facilities with specifically identified equipment are available for the pre-term or ill infant needing special care.

Perinatal transmission of AIDS

The possible routes for virus transmission from mother to infant are:

– transplacental passage
– through the birth canal during delivery
– postnatally, via breast milk or close mother-child contact

HIV has been isolated from cervical secretions,[2] suggesting that infection of the infant could occur through the birth canal. Breast milk was implicated as a source of infection in a case report where a woman was transfused with HIV infected blood following delivery of her infant who was then breast-fed for six weeks.[3]

Current data favours the first route of transmission, suggesting that perinatal HIV infection is congenital. Where pregnancies have been terminated at 15 and 20 weeks, evidence of HIV infection was found in foetal tissue.[4,5] Lapointe *et al*[6] reported on an infant delivered by caesarean section at 28 weeks gestation to a mother with terminal AIDS. Because of its prematurity, the infant died at 28 days of age, having had no post-delivery contact with its mother, and HIV antigen was found in the infant's thymus.

While it is clear that intra-uterine transmission does occur, the present literature does not identify the exact risk of virus transmission from an infected mother to her infant. American studies quote 30 per cent to 50 per cent but these, as already mentioned, concentrate on the severe end of the spectrum, mainly on mothers who have already delivered infants with AIDS. HIV positive but asymptomatic mothers may not have such a high risk of transmission to the infant. Careful follow-up of all pregnant women who are seropositive will also enable definitive guidelines to be issued on the mode of delivery and on breast-feeding. The evidence presented so far, that perinatal HIV infection occurs *in utero*, would suggest that the mode of delivery played little or no part in transmission of virus. The single anecdote[3] implicating breast milk has led to the current advice against breast-feeding. Unless more research emerges to support this advice, there could be dire consequences for infants in developing countries.

Spectrum of HIV infection

Reports which document the clinical manifestations and immunological abnormalities of paediatric HIV infection have concentrated on the more severely affected infants.[7,8,9,10] The mortality of children with AIDS is high, but the ultimate progress of less severely affected children, or asymptomatic children, is unknown.

Table 1 lists the spectrum of HIV infection in children. Three quarters of the children with HIV disease present with non-specific findings in the early stages, but these are nevertheless symptoms of the disease. The Centers for Disease Control in Atlanta, Georgia, has now proposed a new classification of HIV disease in children:

1 the indeterminate group (P-O), that is children aged less than 15 months who have been perinatally exposed, and, because antibody testing is so unhelpful, their infection status is indeterminate

2 children who are 'infected but asymptomatic' (P-1) that is, have no symptoms at all and are healthy carriers. Healthy carriers can be subdivided:
a) those with normal immune function and
b) those with abnormal immune function such as raised immunoglobulin levels, low T4 or white cell count
c) children whose immune function has not been tested

3 'symptomatic' children (P2)
a) those with non-specific symptoms in the early stages of the disease (see Table 1):
– failure to thrive
– generalised lymphadenopathy
– unexplained fever
– enlarged liver and spleen
– diarrhoea
b) those with the more specific signs or symptoms of *progressive neurological disease*, manifested by regression in developmental milestones or in intellect of a child who previously has developed normally. Initially the child may be a little floppy and have abnormalities in gait, then progress to spastic quadriparesis
c) those with the specific disease *lymphoid interstitial pneumonitis*, a kind of lung complaint which differs from pneumocystis in that it is not an opportunistic infection. There are no pathogens grown. This is

peculiar to paediatric HIV disease and has a separate classification in itself

d) those with *recurrent protracted bacterial infections* that could vary from simple upper respiratory tract sepsis (purulent discharge from the ears or nose), recurrent meningitis, recurrent pneumonia or internal organ abscesses

e) those with secondary cancers (rare) or other conditions such as cardiomyopathy, hepatitis, and renal involvement.

Table 1

Spectrum of paediatric HIV infection

1	Non-specific findings	unexplained fever failure to thrive generalised lymphadenopathy parotitis hepatosplenomegaly recurrent diarrhoea eczema persistent candidal infection
2	Lymphoid interstitial pneumonitis	
3	Progressive neurological disease	
4	Recurrent infections	bacterial viral fungal
5	HTLV III embryopathy	
6	Acute glandular-fever-like illness	
7	Opportunistic infections	
8	Laboratory abnormalities	unexplained anaemia thrombocytopaenia polyclonal hypergammaglobulinaemia altered lymphocyte function
9	Secondary malignancies	
10	Others	hepatitis nephropathy cardiomyopathy

Definition of HIV infection

Detection of HIV antibody in an adult or older child is a sensitive and specific indicator of HIV infection, since in the majority of such patients virus culture is positive. A factor which clouds the definition of HIV infection in infants is the presence of passively transferred maternal antibody. The usefulness of a positive antibody test in young infants is thus limited. Although the Edinburgh experience is that infants lose maternal antibody from 9 – 12 months of age, other centres have reported persistence of antibody up to 15 months of age. Therefore it can be argued that the only definitive evidence for infection in a young baby is the identification of HIV in blood or other tissues. At present in the United Kingdom, the low sensitivity of culture systems may mean that a negative virus culture does not necessarily exclude infection.

If virus is to be isolated or cultured from an asymptomatic adult, most laboratories like to deal with 50ml blood, from which there is a 60 per cent chance of a positive result. From infants I send 5ml blood, and the sensitivity of the test is thereby diminished tenfold. Until a more sensitive test is available, careful documentation of clinical signs and immunological abnormalities in all infants born to infected mothers will allow early identification of disease. Antigen testing has now been tried in adults, but the difficulty with children is that we do not know when to expect to find antigen in the blood of each individual child. Nor do we know whether the presence of maternal antibody masks the antigen test.

Routine surveillance in the community

With the setting up of an open-access screening and counselling clinic at the City Hospital in October 1985, HIV seropositive pregnant women were identified. By December 1985, seven infants had been born, necessitating the co-ordination of paediatric surveillance. In January 1986, the paediatric clinic described at the beginning of this paper was established specifically for at-risk infants and their families. To date, 40 families have been enrolled in this clinic. Thirty infants were born to 29 seropositive women. The aims of the paediatric follow-up are:

– to define the risk of virus transmission from the asymptomatic HIV seropositive carrier mother to her infant
– to determine the age of onset of signs and symptoms in the infected

infants, and to study the natural history of HIV disease in infants
– to assess if any co-factors, such as maternal health during pregnancy, mode of delivery and breast-feeding affect the outcome of HIV disease

Community care, including substitute parent care

Where possible, the natural parents are encouraged to look after their infants. However, the haphazard lifestyle led by some parents who continue to abuse drugs means that alternative care has to be sought. It is therefore important for each local authority to prepare all foster parents for the care of HIV seropositive infants. Foster parents have to be told that, wherever possible, they will be informed of the child's HIV status. They should, however, adopt good hygiene practices for all children who come under their care as it is not always possible to identify the HIV status of every child.

The Lothian Region Social Work Department has done pioneering work in preparing foster families to cope with infants born to HIV seropositive women (see Chapter 4). Initially, seminars were held for all foster carers, where basic facts were given on AIDS, transmission of the virus and the low risks during casual contact. Again, general good hygiene practices were emphasised. Specific issues that foster parents must be alerted to are the uncertain outlook for the child, and the assumption that such a child is infected. This means a potentially depressed immune system, so that trivial illnesses have to be treated promptly, and immunisation procedures have to be modified. Where symptoms of HIV disease occur, the child should not be given oral polio, measles, mumps, rubella or BCG vaccination. Following significant exposure to measles or chicken-pox, hyperimmune gammaglobulin should be administered. Inactivated polio vaccine along with diphtheria, tetanus and pertussis can be given. In the asymptomatic carrier, there is a risk of oral polio vaccine being excreted and transmitted to family members who may be immuno-suppressed. Therefore children with asymptomatic HIV infection who are living with infected adults should not be given oral polio vaccine. Measles, mumps and rubella vaccines are now considered safe for asymptomatic children, although their response to immunisation should be closely monitored.

So far, three HIV seropositive infants have been placed successfully in foster care, with a good back-up facility provided by trained nursery nurses willing to give respite care to the foster parents when appropriate. Plans are now in hand for the future of the fostered children, with one couple positively wishing to adopt.

To test or not to test

The clinic has had several referrals from the Social Work Department concerning children and infants where the parents' lifestyles may have involved risks of HIV infection. The usual assumption is that a negative test result will reassure foster parents. While a positive HIV antibody test in an adult usually means past infection, the same cannot be stated for a young infant. As previously mentioned, maternal HIV antibody crosses the placenta and it could take up to 15 months for the infant to clear maternal antibody. By the same reasoning, all infants born to HIV seropositive women will be seropositive due to passively transferred maternal antibody.

I would therefore recommend that, where possible, the mother should be sought for counselling, so that her exact risk can be ascertained. If considered appropriate, the test can then be offered to her. A positive test in the mother means that the infant will have maternal antibody, which may persist till up to 15 months of age. An antibody test in such an infant would be unhelpful in determining the infant's infection status. More detailed tests such as antigen testing or virus culture are at present not readily available nor are they, as I have already indicated, reliable in infants.

Very often the mother is unavailable for testing, and the infant is referred. Careful physical examination, including documentation of growth and development, may reveal signs and symptoms of existing HIV disease. In the absence of any clinical clues, the temptation is to send blood off for HIV antibody. Unless the paediatrician is knowledgeable about the difficulties of interpreting the result, the carers could be lulled into a false sense of security. There have been reports of infants who are HIV antibody negative but where the virus has been grown from lymphocytes.

More sophisticated diagnostic tests are needed to define HIV infection in infants and young children. Also, HIV antibody production in infants is not well understood. If the infant was infected *in utero*, his or her immune system may be so damaged as to be unable to produce antibodies to HIV. Also, if viral genetic material is incorporated into the infant, will his or her immune system recognise HIV material as being foreign and produce antibodies to it?

Until more is known about the pattern of HIV antibody production in infants, the definite diagnosis of HIV infection in perinatally exposed infants under 15 months is extremely difficult. In terms of foster care, the foster parents have to be reassured of the extremely unlikely risk to themselves, if they practise high standards of hygiene. For prospective adopters, it may mean delaying placement if the infant's HIV status has to be guaranteed. This could mean a long wait for the infant who has been perinatally exposed to HIV infection.

The future

Figure 1 attempts to predict the outcome of infants born to HIV seropositive women. Until more is known about the risk of virus transmission from mother to infant, no exact percentages can be quoted. It is not unreasonable to expect that some infants will have escaped HIV infection, but infants will need to be monitored for up to five years before they can be declared free from infection.

Figure 1

The future

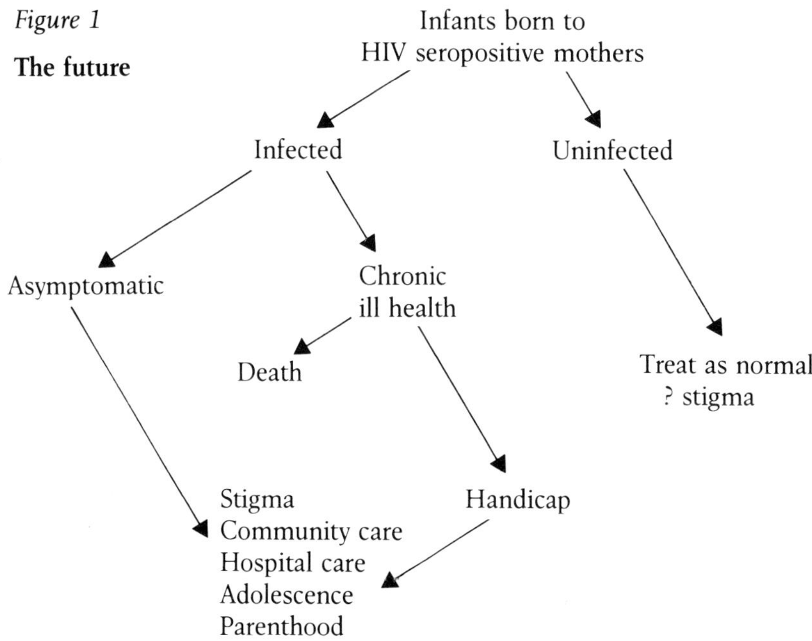

The infected child

Asymptomatic carrier

A proportion of infected children will remain asymptomatic although they are infectious. They and their families need help in living with the stigma and social isolation brought on by being HIV seropositive. It is likely that the child would have been infected through the mother so that at least one, if not both, parents will also be infected. Other children in the household may or may not be similarly affected but will certainly require counselling and support.

The young child with asymptomatic HIV infection should be allowed to lead a normal life. This involves attending school and taking part in all activities. The rights of the child and family to confidentiality must be respected, and this could mean the family choosing not to disclose the child's HIV status to any member of the social work, health care or teaching staff. As clear evidence is emerging that HIV infection is not transmitted through casual contact at the day-care, school or work setting, it could be argued that teachers and schoolmates do not need to know. The fear of being stigmatised, or of other children being withdrawn from the school, will understandably lead to several HIV affected families not disclosing that information.

It is therefore imperative that children and staff at school are educated now on the correct facts surrounding AIDS and the low infectivity of the virus. Current attitudes towards homosexuality and drug abusers have to be examined. It is hoped that, with better understanding, the public will recognise HIV infection as being everybody's problem and will treat infected individuals with sensitivity and sympathy. Education about HIV infection should start early in the school career, and should never be done in isolation without information on health and hygiene, social responsibilities and sex education. Every teacher should be well enough informed about these topics to be able to answer children's questions appropriately, whenever they may arise. (See also Chapter 6 on the role of education.)

Healthy carriers, when approaching adolescence, will have to be counselled on the implications of their disease. This has to start with healthy living and avoidance of activities such as intravenous drug abuse, which will contribute to the development of full-blown AIDS. Adolescents will require support when embarking on relationships with the opposite sex and should be encouraged to adopt a responsible attitude. They may also feel anger towards their parent, who will be blamed for their HIV status, fear about their own future and guilt that they might be responsible for passing the infection to their partner or offspring. With the adoption of safer sex practices there will also come the realisation that they will never be able to have children.

The symptomatic child

Chronic ill-health The incubation period of HIV in children is believed to be shorter than that reported in adults, although the time of onset of signs and symptoms is as yet undefined. Current experience, mainly from symptomatic cases in America, indicate that about 50 per cent of children were diagnosed as having AIDS during the first year of life; and 82 per cent by three years of age. It must be stressed that these cases represent severely-affected children with end-stage disease. Prior to the diagnosis of AIDS, many children will present with chronic ill-health. Infants and young children with HIV infection may have recurrent severe infections, protracted diarrhoea, failure to gain weight as well as neurological complications necessitating recurrent hospitalisations. While the diarrhoea may be difficult to treat, the debilitated child will require medical and nursing care because of dehydration and malnutrition. Regular intravenous infusions of immunoglobulin have been shown to alleviate recurrent infections.

Neurological complications HIV disease of the brain is now well documented in adults as well as children. The neurological involvement is usually progressive, with loss of developmental milestones or intellectual ability, impaired brain growth and motor deficits. As already stated, the affected child could end up with spastic quadriparesis, together with loss of intellect. Such children will make demands on facilities for handicapped children which are already stretched at present. Where one or other parent is affected and ill, alternative care arrangements will be required for the child. This could involve placement with a family or in an institution. Either choice demands that carers are able to take on the added strains of a dementing, physically disabled child with a limited lifespan.

Preparing children for death Children who are old enough will start to ask questions about their future and about the effects of HIV disease on their life, especially if they have had several hospital admissions and endured painful treatments. The majority of adults feel uncomfortable when faced with the question 'Am I going to die?' from a child. Those looking after ill children will need to be prepared for such questions and be able to answer them truthfully, appropriately and with sympathy. The present state of knowledge is that no cure is effective against HIV although some aspects of the disease, for example infection and malnutrition, can be treated.

At some stage, when all therapy has failed, the carers may wish to take the child home for terminal care. Although such a wish has to be respected, the carers must also consider the effects on the other members of the family when a terminally ill child is nursed at home. We have to remember that HIV disease is a disease of the family unit. In many cases the child will be diagnosed first, then the mother and other members of the close family, who may become ill simultaneously. In such cases, the stress inflicted on other relatives can be very severe.

Bereavement support for the family Parents, siblings, members of the wider family and staff will all need to be supported following the death of the child. Feelings of relief, guilt, anger and fear may be very real, especially if any of the family members are similarly infected. Referral to professionals trained in bereavement counselling may help.

Conclusion

The lack of available cure or vaccine against HIV at present makes it necessary to assume that the mortality and morbidity of HIV sero-positive babies will be high. Planning for their future therefore must include consideration of the worst outcome in terms of ill-health and handicap, so that resources can be planned appropriately. The importance of a multi-disciplinary team approach is highlighted, especially in managing sick children and their families. Current attitudes towards and prejudices against homosexuals and drug abusers will have to change, as these risk activities are rarely directly implicated in paediatric HIV disease. Research into vaccines and cures for HIV must be supported so that the prognosis for infected individuals can be improved.

References

1 Scott G B, Fischl M A and Klimas N 'Mothers of infants with the acquired immunodeficiency syndrome' *JAMA* 1985; 253: 363-6.

2 Vogt M W, Witt D J and Craven D E 'Isolation of HTLV III/LAV from cervical secretions of women at risk for AIDS' *Lancet* 1986; i: 525-7.

3 Ziegler J B, Cooper D A and Johnson R O 'Postnatal transmission of AIDS-related retrovirus from mother to infant' *Lancet* 1985; i: 896-8.

4 Sprecher S, Sonmerknoff G and Puissant F 'Vertical transmission of HIV in 15 week foetus' *Lancet* 1986; ii: 288-9.

5 Jovaisis E, Koch M A and Schafer A 'LAV/HTLV III in 20 week foetus' *Lancet* 1985; ii: 1129.

6 Lapointe N, Michand J and Pekovic D 'Transplacental transmission of HTLV III' *New Engl J Med* 1985; 312: 1125-6.

7 Rubinstein A, Sicklich M and Gupta A 'Acquired immunodeficiency with reversed T4/T8 ratio in infants born to promiscuous and drug addicted mothers' *JAMA* 1983; 249: 1350-6.

8 Scott G B, Buck B E and Leterman J G 'Acquired immunodeficiency syndrome in infants' *New Engl J Med* 1984; 310: 76-81.

9 Marion R W, Wiznia A A and Hutcheon G 'Human T-cell lymphotropic virus type III (HTLV III) embryopathy' *AJDC* 1986; 140: 638-40.

10 Epstein L G, Leroy R and Sharer L R 'Neurological manifestations of human immunodeficiency virus infection' *Paediatrics* 1986; 76: 678-87.

4 Placement of children at risk of HIV infection

Anne Black and Kate Skinner

The very high level of HIV positivity among intravenous drug abusers in Edinburgh has created a particular challenge for Lothian, and the following two papers highlight three aspects of HIV infection: management, training and practice. Experience in Lothian indicates that anyone with responsibility for each of these must interlock with the others if a cohesive and effective service is to be offered.

PART 1: A MANAGER'S PERSPECTIVE
Anne Black

One of the overwhelming impressions in much of the work we have done in Lothian has been the uncertainty surrounding many aspects of AIDS. Knowledge has been growing very rapidly regarding medical and social aspects of the disease and, very importantly, public awareness about the HIV virus and AIDS has been initially sketchy and sensational and then intensive and informative. The challenge in so much of the work we have had to do has been to manage those changes and to ensure that information is absorbed alongside recognition of strong emotions. The placement in substitute care of children who are HIV positive depends on staff being informed, aware and available to carers who need extensive support, information and resources, both practical and emotional.

Existing policies
Our primary task in management was to give staff a supportive framework within which to develop services. In any new situation and challenge the temptation is to feel that a whole set of processes and

---

Anne Black is the Divisional Director in Lothian Regional Council Social Work Department with responsibility for adoption and fostering, and as such is closely concerned with the formation of policy and procedures relating to HIV infection. Kate Skinner, an experienced social worker and formerly a member of the adoption and fostering team, is now AIDS Adviser to the Department.

resources will be required and so we may overlook what we already know and indeed provide within our services.

Lothian already had a clear policy of family placement as the option of choice for most children and particularly for those under 12 years of age. This policy has demanded that carers are recruited, trained and supported to offer care to children presenting a range of often quite special needs. This meant that the families we were in touch with had usually cared for children with emotional or physical handicaps and had frequently worked with parents who had difficulties in co-operating with anyone, let alone someone caring actively and well for their child.

As management, we had to confirm that the basic principles of our substitute family placement services were valid for this new challenge. That meant extending our commitment to developing services for children with special needs to include this new group of usually very young children. We had to engage our carers, who had already met the challenge of special needs children, in considering the similarities and differences in caring for a child at risk of being HIV positive. We decided to release an experienced part-time social worker to study the issues of HIV positivity and to work with managers of our family-finding services to build up a pool of carers willing to look after these children.

Using specialist knowledge

To become conversant with the issues, the primary need was for us to forge very good links with our medical colleagues. That was absolutely vital in those early days and has continued to be so as the months have passed. As discussion unfolded, it became clear that across our Department the level of knowledge about AIDS was extremely variable – from ignorance and misunderstanding to, in the areas of high incidence of drug abuse, workers conversant with the issues who were already facing seropositive clients on their caseloads. The need to engage those workers in helping to develop policy and practice guidelines was sometimes overlooked because managers were tempted to become the experts and key sources of knowledge about all aspects of the problem, which sometimes confused issues. While needing a sound grounding about medical facts and social aspects of HIV infection and AIDS, managers must retain a sense of perspective and be prepared to use other staff for much of the detailed planning.

Staff attitudes

The initial months also faced managers with a growing realisation that staff were anxious for their personal safety. Managers had to retain a balance between their responsibilities to deliver social work services in their area and to protect staff from unnecessary health or safety risks. Their fears led some social workers to say that they would not visit certain high-risk families. If this was the reaction within our Department, we had every reason to believe that it would be replicated in our carers. In a strange way this helped to inform our strategy of giving appropriately detailed information to all carers who expressed an initial interest in helping to care for HIV positive children. One important preparatory aspect of building up a small number of carers for HIV positive children was to allow them time to make considered decisions for themselves as a family. It was tempting, in the anxiety about finding places, to want to see carers ready for action. This temptation had to be resisted and workers had to trust the families to make the decisions once the foundation of good information and counselling had been laid. (Kate Skinner discusses in the following paper the detail of our training and information programmes.)

Mobilising resources

Senior managers in Lothian decided to establish a small Advisory AIDS Group of senior operational, training and personnel staff. Here again management must recognise that it cannot be expert in every aspect of its services, and groups like this should include representation from workers dealing with at-risk clients and carers. In Lothian this group was responsible for developing guidelines for staff involved with HIV positive clients and for receiving issues for debate from social workers and residential staff as they arose. The early issues were seldom familiar and in the child care field we were seriously concerned about whether we could rely on our current pool of carers to produce enough good placements for children at risk of HIV. We were advised initially that we might need to find placements in care for 50 babies of HIV positive mothers within the first two years. Debates about resources led to the establishment of a small group of nursery nurses who could be released from their usual day-care activities to open up a small residential unit for such babies. The knowledge that this unit was available to support family care was invaluable as we realised that babies born to many drug-abusing mothers carried a high risk of being

HIV positive as well as being exposed to inconsistent parenting and a sometimes chaotic lifestyle which increased the likelihood of admission to care.

Confidentiality

Confidentiality remained a major management issue. Again, it is our dual role as service givers and resource users which can cause conflict. Some issues were clear but legal advice was sought to ensure that we had taken the right approach. It is not often that complex central government regulations are welcomed but the Boarding Out Regulations* left no room for doubt about the need for our carers to be informed of a baby's being at risk of being HIV positive if such medical knowledge was available. Telling the carers was the most straightforward – but who else needed to know? What about the parents of other children in the placement? What were their rights when all the current research literature underlined the negligible risk of infection from normal family contact? Faced with decisions on a Friday afternoon, when all such crises emerge, senior managers decided that the risk of withholding this information from parents of other children in the placement was too high and that they should have the right to choose whether their child remained with the carer or was moved to another carer. Since then evidence has enabled us to be more confident that by promoting good sensible hygiene any possible risks are greatly reduced so that children in the same placement are safe from infection.

Other management issues

Another factor which management decided to indicate in guidelines to staff was that a child who was possibly HIV positive should not be placed in a family where there were young children. Initially children under eight were felt to be more vulnerable as they could not fully appreciate the special aspects of caring for a child of an HIV positive mother. In the intervening months we have revised our thinking and now look at each situation as it arises, with no absolute embargo on placements where there are other young children. But the incontrovertible fact is that caring for such a child needs time, energy and

---

*The *Boarding Out and Fostering of Children (Scotland) Regulations 1985* require that background information about children must be given to substitute parents.

stamina. The family's capacity to cope with this, given its own circumstances and constellation, must be carefully assessed.

Managers must also address the question of availability of a range of resources to carers – we so often think of foster parents of babies as being almost 'in pocket' with fostering allowances, but high costs for consistent warmth, travel, babysitting, etc, all become factors when caring for a baby at risk of HIV. Managers need to be sensitive to this and to be prepared to process special payments.

Children with special needs must have plans made for their future, however uncertain that future may be. Routes for permanence and reviews of progress must be carefully monitored and managers must keep abreast of the particular issues provoked by long-term planning, thus ensuring that policy continues to keep up with new practice issues.

As knowledge has developed, many of these issues have become more complex rather than clearer. The question of whether there should be screening of all babies coming into care or only those where a parent is believed to be at risk of infection is one of the most contentious. The difficulty of ascertaining virus status in the child's own right compounds the problems of planning for children in care. The uncertainties provoked may debilitate carers rather than reassure them. The right of the mother to refuse to undergo tests remains and our right to impose testing on a child needs to be debated. So far we are not seeking to test mothers and babies routinely but are aware of the real need to keep this under close review. Managers must remain sensitive to the dilemmas that screening can bring and be prepared to keep the lines open for debate as knowledge and practice wisdom grows.

PART II: TRAINING AND PRACTICE ISSUES

Kate Skinner

Preparation of foster families

In this paper I discuss the various issues concerning the placement of children of mothers who are, or are likely to be, HIV positive. As Dr Mok has explained in her paper, it is impossible to establish until at least the second year whether the children themselves are seropositive, so they can be described as being 'at risk of HIV positivity'. In order to avoid cumbersome repetition, I shall refer to these children simply as 'at risk'.

With the benefit of hindsight, I am now quite clear that there are no short cuts in providing substitute family care for at-risk children. We began with two babies in urgent need of placement and it was anxiety about the damage to them of prolonged hospital care which generated the energy to embark on what has proved to be a long and time-consuming piece of work. At that time, some of our medical colleagues were advising us, from experience in the USA, that we would be unable to place these children.

Our initial approaches to families were made via their liaison social workers, who were asked to consider families in the light of the information we possessed, which was that the virus was much more difficult to transmit than was conveyed by the press. Alongside this was the indication that the outlook for these babies was very poor indeed. Our view was that we should make available to families the information and knowledge that we ourselves had, including the difficulties and uncertainties, and support them in deciding for themselves whether or not they could offer to care for an at-risk child. We believe that when a family's offer of substitute care has been investigated and accepted by an agency and the agency has subsequently given them full information about the child, including the risks involved in caring for him or her, the ultimate responsibility as to whether or not they accept the child rests with the substitute parents. Circumstances may arise after placement to alter this balance of responsibility, and I return to this issue later in this paper.

Families were asked if they would be prepared to hear more about AIDS and HIV infection and, if they agreed, a meeting was arranged between myself and their liaison worker to explore some of the issues. Next, a further session was arranged with Dr Mok, the Consultant Paediatrician with special responsibility for monitoring the progress of these babies in Lothian. She gave the families as much medical information about the disease as possible, again including the uncertainties. Several of these sessions included teenage or adult family members who wanted to hear the information for themselves. My own experience of trying to learn about and understand AIDS and HIV infection led me to believe that people needed time to assimilate the facts and to allow their significance to emerge, so a short time was allowed between these meetings. A follow-up session between the family and their own worker was then arranged and, interestingly, the first three families to express interest all subsequently offered placements for at-risk children.

An additional spur to me was the help I received from a foster family from outside our own area who were caring for Danny, a child already showing the symptoms of AIDS. They were very open about their feelings on learning about Danny's illness and its implications for their daily lives.

The natural mothers of all of these children have been drug abusers and the preparation of carers has included some information about this problem. Families have needed to explore and air their views about drug abuse in general and about the responsibility that these parents must bear if the virus is passed on to their children. The children are usually seen by carers as 'innocent victims' of HIV infection.

The families who have offered to take HIV positive children have had further opportunities to explore this area in more detail, but do not seem to have found it a major problem. Time was also spent on preparing them to co-operate with and work alongside the natural parents. Contact between the foster family and natural family has been offered for each child. In one case visits were only by the maternal grandparents, in another a number of visits were made to parents in prison and, in a third, there were very frequent visits to the foster home by both parents and siblings. Despite considerable potential for difficulty, all concerned have coped very well.

When we first approached families to take at-risk children, our belief was that of those children born with their mother's antibodies to the virus, a quarter would remain HIV positive at six months of age. Of these, half would remain as carriers of the virus, probably for all of their childhood and adult lives. The other half of the babies would go on to develop the disease, probably at around a year old, and would die very young, probably before they reached the age of four. Our information about the outlook has changed slightly but it remains very uncertain indeed.

This prognosis shocked families, but it also provoked the feeling that the children should receive the very best that family care could provide. This determination has clearly fuelled the foster families to deal with the stresses and strains of these placements. They do have to work at remembering the uncertain prognosis as they all prefer to take, in the main, a day-to-day approach to caring for the children. However, the frequency of medical checks and their knowledge about the disease with its varied presentation and onset helps to alert them to the appearance of signs and symptoms, hence they are aware of the dangers of complacency. Each family deals with its pain about the child's future in its own way. Having access to specialised social work help has been important to them, but they have received also more intimate support from their own social worker and the child's social worker.

The first two babies were placed with their families early in 1986 and are still in placement, so we have had the opportunity of continuing to work with them, learning as we go along.

Back-up and support

Very early on, one of the foster parents identified several strands to her need for support. One was the need for a regular break – as a way of preventing a build-up of pressure. So I arranged for an experienced and competent childminder to offer weekly relief, thus enabling the foster mother to have time off for a swim. This family also felt the need to share full knowledge about the child with a close friend who would be a personal ally and would give support through whatever lay ahead. This support was quite different and separate from that offered by the various professionals involved. Our enhanced fostering payment scheme, which is based on the presence of complexities in the child's family background or behaviour, permitted payment of double the usual allowances to these foster families.

In another foster family, an undertaking to make acceptable arrangements for the baby to be cared for while they were on holiday proved to be very significant. The holiday placement was arranged and went very smoothly indeed.

In a complex new situation like this one, where roles among the professionals are unclear and changing, tolerance and goodwill have kept relationships constructive and minimised difficulties. The importance of this cannot be over-emphasised.

Experience of fostering has shown that, occasionally, circumstances within the foster parent's own family precipitate the need for a change in placement, temporary or otherwise. The hospital ward which initially cared for the first at-risk children offered emergency respite care for these parents on demand. Although not used, the availability of this service helped to minimise any isolation the families might have felt. A group of nursery nurses has subsequently been trained and prepared to augment foster families should this be required in order to avoid inappropriate hospital admission or change in placement.

Mutual support among the foster families has proved to be most valuable. Our last meeting involved six families (one from outside our area), five of whom brought their foster children with them. This was a very potent and moving meeting, which I know I shall never forget. One of the children has already been adopted by his former foster family, and two more families hope to adopt their foster children. Another child is waiting for a permanent family, while another, whose prognosis is not good, is already ill. All the adults experienced the meeting as both a happy and sad occasion. They also emphasised the importance of acknowledging painful areas in the children's lives and how contact with each other helps them to maintain this. Sharing experience has also helped the families to protect themselves from the insensitivity of others about it, often with the aid of their sense of humour.

Training for foster families

Having placed the first two children with foster families, we turned our attention to giving information to all our other carers, some of whom were becoming anxious. Our first training model involved a number of seminars, for a maximum of 40 people. For the first series Dr Mok made a brief medical input but subsequently I took this role myself, in close consultation with her. However, much of the important material was dealt with by responding to families' questions. Hearing about and responding to the concerns of the families proved to be a key to allaying fears and building confidence about HIV infection and its implications.

In these sessions I developed the issues concerning fostering and social work practice. An important part of our training strategy was helping families to see the need to improve their hygiene for *all* children in their care, given that it is quite possible for an unidentified HIV positive child to be placed with them without our knowledge. An invaluable tool in these sessions was a video we made with the family from outside our area who was fostering Danny, a child with AIDS. This took the form of an interview highlighting issues about acceptance of the diagnosis of HIV infection by the family and its implications for neighbours, friends and the local Mother and Toddler Group, and to stress the simple but important preventive measures needed. This video has been very powerful in conveying how quite ordinary people have managed to face up to the complex and painful issues involved.

Notes of guidance to carers were written and distributed to foster families at the training sessions as a reminder of the content. These comprised simple details about the disease and its development in children, and the preventive measures advocated by the Social Work Department.

Following these sessions – about 20 in all – 12 families came forward willing to offer placements to at-risk children. Each family was followed up in a similar way to the initial group and, after discussion, added to the pool. We see these families as potentially available for at-risk children, while not restricting placements with them solely to this group.

We have also prepared and trained a foster parent who is willing to offer an emergency placement solely for a young child who is HIV positive.

Practice issues arising from our experience so far

The delicate issue of confidentiality has led us to advise our carers that only those people who *have* to know (ie health visitor and family doctor) should be told about the presence of an at-risk child in the family. However, we know that practice has varied among our families and we have to report that so far there have been no adverse reactions from neighbours, playgroups etc. It does, however, remain a significant issue.

Who should know about the placement of an HIV positive child? What about the parents of other foster children? What about the social workers for other foster children? As our view is that other children are *not* at risk from the presence in a family of a child at risk, we feel that we do not need to advise other parents. This applies also to nurseries and schools. However, we have advised all parents in our own children's centres that at some point their children may come into contact with an HIV positive child while at the centre. This, we believe, should avoid any unnecessary and damaging stigmatising of particular children.

Should these children be placed in families where there are other young children? We are assured that group care for them is permissable so long as reasonable, basic hygiene is practised, so why not? We have opted for a policy that we should minimise the complexities in placements where we can, and where we have a choice.

I stated earlier that substitute parents carry responsibility on behalf of their family for assessing and accepting the risks involved in caring for an at-risk child, the agency's responsibility at that stage being to ensure that they are given full information and time in which to make a considered decision. After placement, however, three factors are brought to bear on the situation. First, the family is likely to become deeply attached to the child; second, having embarked upon a difficult task they will usually be keen to see it through to its conclusion; and third, the agency workers are usually in a better position than the family to keep abreast of recent developments in the field of HIV infection and its transmission. When, for instance, a child with open skin lesions was found to be at risk of infection, his substitute parents wanted to continue to care for him. They had in a very short time become attached to him and also felt that, by allowing his removal, they would betray their commitment to him as foster parents. Our keen awareness of the increased risks presented to all members of the family by the skin lesions prompted us to assume greater responsibility here and the child was removed, to become the only child placed so far in the professional unit mentioned earlier. This situation demonstrates clearly the balance that the placing agency must maintain at all times between, on the one hand, reassurance (against the rumours that are rife in the community) that the risk of transmission through family contact is infinitessimal and, on the other hand, constant vigilance regarding the risks that clearly do exist.

All of the children placed so far, five in Lothian and two in another area, have been in short-term placements while plans are made for their future. In three out of the seven placements, however, the families have shown an interest in adopting their foster child. This is far too small a number to be statistically significant, but we have noted that in each case bonding and commitment between family and child is exceptionally strong.

PART III: CONCLUSIONS RELATING TO BOTH MANAGEMENT AND PRACTICE

The placement of at-risk children in substitute care will continue to challenge departments as our knowledge and experience develops.

New issues emerge as we move from temporary care to permanency planning.

The partnership between medical staff, substitute parents and social work staff must continue to underpin these placements. Opportunities for training, education and support for special carers must continue to be provided. Skills and resources to support carers faced with a terminally ill child must be developed. Again, while we are not totally unfamiliar with these needs, we as managers must recognise that workers will require time and skill in order to support these special placements. Very importantly, workers themselves will need support to enable them to cope with the many emotional stresses inevitably brought about by this new area of work.

The two parts of this chapter attempt to outline some of the problems we have tackled in the time we have been working in this area. We cannot claim to be experts or that the steps we have taken would be right for all circumstances. We hope that, by making our experience available, others will try to build on it and develop their own services for children who bear this new and distressing burden.

5 AIDS: some legal implications for children

Richard White

This paper will examine:

a) the law in England and Wales relating to children who are in care or who may be brought into care as a result of contact with the AIDS virus
b) application of the law to particular groups of children
   - adolescent children in care
   - children to be fostered or adopted or in placement
   - the sexually abused child
c) confidentiality

The law

It is important to remember that there is a legal framework within which local authorities are required to take decisions.

Care proceedings

Under the Children and Young Persons Act 1969 (CYPA), section 2(1), if *'a local authority receive information suggesting that there are grounds for bringing care proceedings in respect of a child (under 14 years) or young person (14 – 17 years) . . . it shall be the duty of the authority to cause enquiries to be made . . .'* and in section 2(2) *'if it appears to a local authority that there are grounds for bringing care proceedings . . . it shall be the duty of the authority to exercise their power to bring care proceedings, unless they are satisfied that it is neither in his interest nor the public interest to do so . . .'.*

Where a child is HIV seropositive or is suffering from the AIDS disease, there is every reason to believe that the grounds for care

---

Richard White is a solicitor practising in family law and is the Editor of Clarke, Hall and Morrison: the law relating to children and young persons. *He is the joint author of several publications on child care law and is a former chairman of the British Association for the Study and Prevention of Child Abuse and Neglect.*

proceedings may be satisfied, depending on the circumstances in which the infection was acquired. If a child or young person is at risk of acquiring the disease, the ground may also be satisfied.

The relevant grounds are (under CYPA section 1(2)) that '*any of the following conditions is satisfied with respect to the child*
a) his proper development is being avoidably prevented or neglected or his health is being avoidably impaired or neglected or he is being ill treated or . . .
b) he is exposed to moral danger . . .
c) and that he is in need of care or control which he is unlikely to receive unless the court makes an order . . .'.
It will be apparent that if a young person is having a relationship with an older person or is promiscuous, he or she may be in moral danger. The possibility of a sexual partner being seropositive or having AIDS inevitably heightens the risks for the young person and perhaps makes it more likely that the court would be satisfied that the child is in need of care or control.

Recent case law has established that the grounds for care proceedings can be satisfied where the impairment of health was caused by behaviour of the parent before the child's birth, provided that behaviour was avoidable and provided that the child was in need of care and control at the time of the proceedings (Re D (A Minor) [1987] 1 FLR 422). Thus it could be that the child of a mother who passes the virus through the foetus might properly be the subject of care proceedings, because of the mother's promiscuous behaviour or ill-advised sexual behaviour. Proceedings might also be considered in respect of a child whose mother has AIDS and who refused advice not to breast-feed. Grounds might also arise where the parent became incapable of caring adequately because of the advent of the disease.

Clearly at present there are difficulties in establishing evidence in these circumstances. Medical experts are unable to predict whether a baby who is HIV positive will remain so, because he or she could lose the mother's antibodies during the first two years of life. Tests being developed may produce better evidence in due course.

A parent may further question whether the health of a child who is seropositive is being impaired, since it is not clear at that stage what actual impairment has occurred. New grounds proposed in the White Paper (The Law on Child Care and Family Services, Cm 62) which require 'evidence of harm or likely harm, attributable to the absence of a reasonable standard of parental care' do not appear to resolve this point. This proposal might provide a basis for proceedings in respect of a neonate whom the mother insists on breast-feeding, although the evidence of transmission of the virus by that route is also thin.

In difficult cases such as may be presented by AIDS, it may be preferable to use wardship, so that the wider powers of the High Court are available to give directions as to the future of the child and to ensure that there is no publicity that might be detrimental to the child.

Statutory duty of care

Under the Child Care Act 1980 (CCA), section 18(1),

'In reaching any decision relating to a child in their care, a local authority shall give first consideration to the need to safeguard and promote the welfare of the child throughout his childhood; and shall so far as practicable ascertain the wishes and feelings of the child regarding the decision and give due consideration to them, having regard to his age and understanding'.

This is subject to sub-section (3), which states

'If it appears to a local authority that it is necessary for the purpose of protecting members of the public, to exercise their powers in relation to a particular child in their care in a manner which may not be consistent with their duty under ss(1), the authority may notwithstanding that duty act in that manner'.

In pursuance of the duty in sub-section (1) the local authority will normally be obliged to act in the child's best interests and do everything it can to ensure that proper steps are taken for his or her welfare. This will include placing the child in surroundings which will best promote their upbringing. Unless the child requires hospitalisation, this will often mean that the child will be placed in a substitute family.

There may be a conflict of interest in the case of an older child, if the duty to the public applies. In certain circumstances, where it becomes necessary for an authority to restrict the liberty of a child for more than 72 hours, it may have to use its powers under the Secure Accommodation Regulations 1983 to obtain authority from the juvenile court for a longer period of detention.

Exercise of parental rights and duties

It should be remembered that if a child is in care under CYPA or CCA (where parental rights have also been assumed under that act) the local authority has wide powers in respect of the child, which include the exercise of medical consents. The Gillick case suggests there may be some limitation on this in respect of older children who are capable of forming a mature view of their situation, but it remains unclear precisely what powers an authority has to control an older child.

Application of the law to particular groups of children

Adolescents in care

The particular difficulty with this age group in relation to HIV infection is that they are most likely to be sexually active. They will also include children who are likely to or have absconded. Additionally this age group is the most likely to be living in residential accommodation and in the company of other, similar, children.

a) Should a child who has absconded or is thought to have engaged in a 'risky' relationship be
i) offered a test? (This would appear to depend on general principles related to counselling.)
ii) required to submit to a test? (There was general agreement among those present at the seminar that it would be an inappropriate use of parental authority to require a child to take a test, or to authorise a test where blood has been taken for other reasons.)

b) Should a child who is known to be at risk but not known to be affected be treated as affected?

c) What precautions should be taken for the safety of and what knowledge should be given to
i) other children
ii) staff
in respect of a child who is known to be promiscuous or violent?
It has to be accepted that adolescents in care are in a high-risk group. There should be a general policy in all child care agencies to ensure a high standard of health education including an understanding of sexually transmitted diseases and diseases transmitted by infection of blood. Young people would then be alerted to the risks.

One outstanding issue concerns the duty of an authority with a seropositive child in its care towards another child in its care who is having or may be having a sexual relationship with the first child. There are conflicting duties of confidence to the first child and to the care of the second. This writer would resolve those in favour of the second child being informed about the condition of the first.

Children fostered or placed for adoption

There are no requirements at present for a medical examination on the admission of a child to care, although as a matter of local practice most authorities carry out a 'freedom from infection' test. This would not reveal the presence of HIV.

If a child is fostered, the Boarding Out of Children Regulations 1955 (England and Wales) set minimum limits. Regulation 6 states that '*Except in an emergency, a child shall not be boarded out with foster parents unless he has within three months before being placed with them been examined by a duly qualified medical practitioner and the practitioner has made a written report on the physical health and mental condition of the child.*' Regulation 7 has further requirements after boarding out.

It is at least arguable that these regulations cover a test for HIV, since the condition relates to the physical health of the child. However, as argued above, a child should not be required to be tested.

There is no provision in the Boarding Out Regulations 1955 for England and Wales (as there is in Scotland), requiring transmission of health information to foster parents. If there is definite information available to the authority, good practice indicates that this should also be made available to a foster parent and the Regulations should be amended to provide for this, not least because it will be important to track the child's health progress. If information is not available, foster parents should in any event be advised to use high standards of hygiene and should be told about the child's social background, as this may indicate that the child is in a high-risk group.

If a child is being considered for adoption, more rigorous requirements are set out in the Adoption Agencies Regulations 1983. By regulation 7, the adoption agency must set up a case record and place on it information obtained by virtue of that regulation. This information includes particulars of the parents and child set out in a Schedule and a written medical report dealing with matters specified in the Schedule. The agency shall also '*arrange such other examinations and screening procedures of and tests on the child and, so far as is reasonably practical, his parents, as are recommended by the adoption agency's medical adviser . . .*'. The Schedule refers to '*any special needs in relation to the child's health (whether physical or mental)*' and '*a full health history and examination of the child including details of any serious illness*'. In relation to the parents, including where appropriate the putative father, the report should include '*a family health history, covering the parents, the brothers and sisters (if any) and the other children of the parent with details of any serious physical or mental illness and inherited and congenital disease*' and '*a full obstetric history of the mother, including any problems in the ante-natal, labour and post-natal periods, with the results of any tests carried out during or immediately after pregnancy*'.

Whether information relevant to AIDS or HIV positivity will be discovered through these procedures is uncertain. The mother may not be available or may refuse to be tested. Indeed it is possible that she will be counselled not to take a test. At the seminar it was suggested that a test on the child for HIV at present yields information about the mother rather than about the child, and should therefore not be revealed without her consent, even in a child subject to a care order. However, in my opinion the child is the patient and therefore the information relates to him or her. Information in relation to the mother's health history may exclude any reference to HIV infection. If she has been tested and agrees for the sake of her child to that information being passed to the adoption agency, it should be passed on to prospective adopters, with advice that it is not a conclusive indication of the child's serostatus. There seems to be little purpose in encouraging mothers who wish to place their children for adoption but who are not members of an 'at-risk' group to be tested.

If the child is for some reason tested and found to be seropositive we have seen that this is not conclusive until the child has lost all maternal antibodies. The best advice seems to be that prospective adopters should be told that babies of some parents are at high risk from a number of diseases. They should not expect specific testing for HIV infection.

The adoption agency is obliged by regulation 12 to provide a prospective adopter with, among other things, a health history of the child before the placement. Adopters have a right to such information as is available about a child before taking on responsibility for him or her, so that they can consider the implications for themselves and their family. They may, for example, be prevented from taking up residence in certain countries if immigrant testing is introduced.

Sexually abused children

The third category of children who may suffer problems related to HIV is that of sexually abused children, whether by their own family or by a stranger. From the cases we have seen in the courts of multiple abuse across the generations, it is clearly only a matter of time before a child becomes infected in this way. Substitute families caring for such children will have to be carefully chosen for their ability to deal sensitively with the issues and to maintain high standards of hygiene.

The principles for dealing with such cases are the same as for younger children, but there may additionally be specific information about the child's condition.

Confidentiality

The General Medical Council's Code of Professional Conduct states: *'It is a doctor's duty strictly to observe the rule of professional secrecy by refraining from disclosing voluntarily to any third party information about a patient which he has learnt directly or indirectly in his professional capacity as a registered medical practitioner. The death of the patient does not absolve the doctor from this obligation.'* None of the exceptions to this rule would entitle a doctor to inform a third party about the state of his or her patient's health for the protection of the third party. Furthermore, as a result of damaging prejudice in the community, many counsellors at present caution those seeking advice against having the test for fear of the implications of the knowledge that they are seropositive. Following the Gillick case a mature child of, say, 15, could require her GP not to tell her parents about her condition.

Applying this to the situation of a child in care, the local authority *in loco parentis* may not be made aware that a child is seropositive. It is therefore in no position to offer protection to other children in its care. In the USA there is a growing body of case law holding an individual responsible for informing a partner that he or she has a sexually transmitted disease ('The initial impact of AIDS on public health law in the United States',*Law and Medicine*, 16 January 1987), and in the UK it has been argued that this could be a criminal offence (*Law Society's Gazette*, 25 March 1987). Could it be argued that a doctor has a duty of disclosure to persons whom he might reasonably contemplate would be affected?

The GMC Code appears at present to place responsibility for disclosure solely with the seropositive person. This can be interpreted as implying that he or she will exercise a sense of responsibility. It is not unsympathetic to the victims to question whether all of them will fulfil that responsibility and this may be especially true of children and young people, who will be frightened. It is difficult to balance the need to protect confidence, thus encouraging affected people to come forward for counselling and treatment, with the need to prevent the spread of the disease by warning possible contacts. The denial of disclosure to certain limited categories of people needs to be more rigorously examined.

6 AIDS – the role of education and its implications for young people

Colin Griffiths

The education approach

Two years ago in the UK, the role of education was still considered to have very little value in informing the public or in tackling the spread of AIDS or HIV infection. The level of anxiety amongst both professionals and public alike was enormous and there were few organised educational strategies for any of the groups most at risk of infection. In the intervening two years, our experience of working with young people in Wales has given us useful guidelines on which to draw when starting to educate groups of young people. First of all, before planning any educational programme at a local level, three questions must be asked:

– why do we need a health education programme?
– how do we disseminate the information?
– what target groups do we need to get the information to?

Why do we need an education programme?

We need an education programme for two reasons:

– to raise awareness and develop basic knowledge about the disease, in an attempt to allay the myths and anxieties that exist
– to try, through provision of information, to modify individual behaviour, in an attempt to limit the spread of HIV infection

How do we disseminate the information?

Direct contact is essential. When discussing AIDS – regardless of which group we are dealing with – many issues and specific questions will be raised, the answers to which always need to be qualified. It is no

---

Colin Griffiths is a neuroscientist. He read for his PhD at St George's Hospital and then worked for five years in the Department of Psychology at Oxford. After two years on the staff of the University of Montreal he returned to the UK in 1985 and initiated the West Glamorgan AIDS Education project before being appointed as Director of the Welsh AIDS Campaign.

use answering, 'you can't' or 'you mustn't': people always ask, 'why?' There must be someone present who is qualified to answer questions like these: no video, film or leaflet used in isolation can cover all the issues raised.

What target groups do we want to get this information to?
Two years ago the target group considered to be most at risk was gay men. Nowadays we recognise that there are different target groups and it is essential to provide specific information to satisfy the needs of each group. General campaigns, which attempt to include different messages for different groups (for example, combining general education to raise awareness with education aimed at modifying behaviour) are less likely to succeed than those targetted specifically at individual groups.

It is essential therefore to select one group and to design a programme appropriate to its needs. What is relevant information for one group will not satisfy the needs of another. It is important too to evaluate any programme – to know that the group of people targetted has understood and has gone out and carried the message further.

Teenagers as the target group
I would now like to deal with one group in particular, that is, teenagers, following a programme I recently organised in South Wales. After negotiation with the local education department it was agreed that I would visit the majority of comprehensive schools in West Glamorgan. The age groups that I would talk to would be fourth, fifth and sixth formers and, in order to get as balanced a view as possible, it was decided that the parents would also be involved. So a programme was organised whereby during the day I spoke to the pupils and in the evening the parents were invited along to hear the same talk and to discuss any issues raised. This gave me the chance to talk to a large selection of the public and also provided an opportunity for feedback.

I decided that the best plan for this group was to set AIDS in the context of sexually transmitted diseases. Many of the pupils had received talks earlier on along these lines and therefore AIDS could be included in the ongoing programme for general health education in the school. Although obviously I mentioned transmission by blood and shared syringes, my main focus was on AIDS as a sexually transmitted disease.

The content of an education programme

Any education programme on AIDS is based, quite simply, on the four main things that people want to know:

– what is AIDS?

– where does it come from? (I do not talk about the genesis of HIV, rather about the problems caused by the virus)

– how is it transmitted?

– why does it affect the particular groups that it does?

It seems safe to assume that nearly everybody has one main concern: that if they get AIDS they will die. So they want to know how they can get it and how they can avoid getting it. That is the basis of a good education programme – it must be kept simple. And, because of the constantly developing state of knowledge, it has to be stressed that the programme is based on the present state of knowledge only.

There has been controversy recently about how explicit a campaign should be. I believe that we have to talk in language that people understand. We can be explicit without being offensive. It is essential to put the message in terms comprehensible to the audience. The point for this group of teenagers was: the greater the number of casual sexual partners they have, the greater the chance of picking up a sexually-transmitted disease, and the same applies to picking up HIV infection.

Teenagers do not want detailed information about the virus. They are not interested. They want to know what it means to *them*. They want something interesting, something relevant. I produced a leaflet for teenagers which is simple but striking (see pages 74 to 77, where the main contents of the leaflet are reproduced). It contains virtually no medical information. This was piloted throughout Wales. I took it to the local prison, to young offenders and to a group who had reading difficulties. I took it here, there and everywhere, to schools and youth groups, and the same message came back: 'Well, it tells us what we should do and what we should not do.' That is the whole point of work with teenagers.

There is an argument that, because the spread of the disease among heterosexuals is still rare, we are creating unnecessary panic. But the figures we have today on AIDS cases (never mind the levels of infection with HIV) are, because of the incubation period, the result of infection contracted three to five years ago. So the number of people in Britain now who will develop AIDS will not be seen for another few years.

Response to the programme

Following the talks to both pupils and parents I allowed plenty of time for questions. The questions asked were extremely varied. From the parents, there were no objections at all to the programme. In fact, most groups of parents commented, 'Surely you should be doing this with the younger age group?'. The type of questions the young people asked astonished me. They get most of their information from the media but are extremely well clued-up. They think about it. No-one should ever think that teenagers are not considering things. For instance, some would come and find me after a meeting of four or five hundred pupils. One fourteen-year-old said, 'After what you told us now, if it is killing off all these white cells that protect us, why can we not replace the white cells? That is what they do in a bone marrow transplant isn't it?'

One of the more amusing questions was 'Is AIDS transmitted by black pudding?' This boy's point was that black pudding is made of blood and AIDS is transmitted by blood. One girl came up to me and said: 'After what you said I talked to two of my friends and, say, we want to go out on Saturday night. How do girls get sheaths if we want to carry them?' They are thinking, and they are putting two and two together. Never underestimate their basic knowledge. We can increase it, but only by direct contact. They need to have someone there to talk to them. They want basic information, aimed at what they want to know and designed to make them think.

One of the difficulties I encountered was the apparent lack of motivation among teenagers for any form of behavioural change. It is still the general opinion among them that AIDS won't happen to them, that there is really no need to cut down on sexual partners because this is still largely a disease of gay men. The necessity of organising widespread education programmes for teenagers is emphasised by this attitude.

Wider issues

This paper has dealt with the educational approach to one group of young people, but other public health issues are equally important. Particularly difficult issues are raised by young children of infected mothers. Such infants frequently come from socially disadvantaged homes. Mothers may be drug abusers and may be sick with AIDS themselves with a short life expectancy. These infants consequently may be cared for by foster or adoptive parents. There is every reason to believe that having an infected foster child in the home is safe for the caretakers, yet the stigma of AIDS may make placement difficult. These problems have been discussed more fully in other papers.

It remains for me to say that, in addition to education programmes designed for teenagers, it is as well to implement now some policies on education programmes for day and residential carers and the families in which infected children may be placed.

7 Conclusions and summary of recommendations

There are at present relatively few children in the UK who are known to be HIV positive compared with the United States and some European countries where the incidence of infection has increased rapidly. This offers us an opportunity to develop strategies which might inhibit widespread transmission of the disease and which could certainly improve the lifestyle of those children who are at high risk of infection. Participants at the BAAF seminar in May 1987 were conscious of this opportunity throughout their deliberations, although sometimes also baffled by the complexity of its implications.

Discussions in the small groups and in the plenary sessions centred on three main issues:

- education and training for all involved
- confidentiality of information regarding HIV status
- the needs of carers

Linking these issues there is a fourth:

- decision-making

This chapter will discuss each of the first three in turn, and will end by drawing up a list of recommendations that we offer for consideration by individual agencies.

Education and training

Why education?

Despite the fact that consumer research by the DHSS indicates that information from the national publicity campaign launched in 1986 has been digested by some members of the public, a distressing degree of ignorance, rumour and prejudice remains. Counteracting this and promoting accurate knowledge among agency staff and substitute parents about HIV infection will enable agencies to plan more effectively for individual children. For instance, reassurance that the virus is not transmitted through ordinary family contact and that it is easily destroyed when outside the body will enable many workers to contemplate family placement for children in their care. So appropriate education programmes are of prime importance in overall agency planning.

Armed with accurate information, agency staff may in turn find opportunities to affect and modify community attitudes, thus eventually ensuring greater support for those caring for at-risk children in the community. Informed media coverage has done much to expand support in the community for those caring for special needs children. Similarly, agencies can encourage participation in responsible programmes about HIV infection.

Reaching the people involved

Two factors are of prime importance in all education programmes, particularly those concerning serious risks to health. These are:

– To be most effective information should first cover facts which are wanted and needed by the target group. Colin Griffiths, in Chapter 6, explains that he deliberately avoids offering extraneous information to teenagers. Contributors at the seminar emphasised that foster parents want details relevant to the day-to-day care of children and to the avoidance of transmission rather than, for instance, precise notes on the origins of the virus.

– Talks, slides and videos are not enough. There must be face-to-face contact with informed educators, either through a series of meetings or a consultation service of some sort.

Participants at the seminar agreed that children in care should not be singled out as a group for special education in this area, but that agencies should ensure that education is available to them either at school or through some group in the community. Carers, however, would have a special role as counsellors, providing informed back-up to a group programme.

Keeping information up to date

Rumours purporting to be fresh information can create new anxieties and set back an education programme several stages. Agency staff need to feel confident that they are being kept informed. This is best done by deploying a member of staff specifically to keep abreast of developments in this field. He or she need not be a manager and may more effectively be someone already known to carers. This worker's duties should include alerting management to the need for refresher education programmes as well as to the need for resources.

Maintaining high standards of hygiene
We have seen in previous chapters that it is impossible at present to identify with any accuracy which children are HIV positive. Carers must recognise the fact that HIV infection may be present at any time and must therefore provide an appropriate standard of care at all times. Ordinary standards of hygiene as recommended by Health Authorities are sufficient protection against transmission of the disease. However, we have to accept that practice has sometimes fallen short of such standards in recent years and serious efforts must be made to re-establish them in day, residential and family care. Practical instructions regarding hygiene should be part of any education programme and a system for monitoring should be set up.

Confidentiality of information relating to HIV status

The medical ethic
The BMA Guidelines concerning HIV status are based on those laid down by the General Medical Council governing the relationship between a doctor and his or her patient. These state that a doctor must not divulge medical information about a patient without consent, and this applies to the result of a test for HIV infection or antibodies. The exceptions to this rule – when the patient's life or the wider community is at risk if the information is not divulged – are not considered to be applicable in law to HIV infection, nor does the law at present allow divulgence of information for the sake of the patient's child. It could be that the situation would change somewhat should a vaccine or a cure for HIV infection become available, but at present the permission of the patient is necessary before a test can be carried out on a child or the result divulged to anyone beyond the tester, unless the child is in care under a Care Order or a Parental Rights and Duties resolution, or is a ward of court. Even in these circumstances, difficulties could arise because a test result at present represents confidential medical information about the mother rather than about the child.

Whether or not to test
It is clear that the present test for antibodies is not reliable in a child under two years, nor is it totally reliable in older children and adults,

since both false negative and false positive results have been obtained. Social information about the child's family (that is, whether or not the mother is a member of an at-risk group) should be weighed against the likelihood of stigmatisation of the child. Testing of the parent is preferable in every case, but we must be aware of the implications of testing and ensure that parents are properly counselled. In the opinion of contributors to the BAAF seminar, testing is not appropriate at present for children whose parents are not members of an at-risk group, and BAAF suggests that very careful thought should be given to a decision regarding the testing of any asymptomatic child in care. In every case the decision whether or not a child should be submitted to a test, or a natural mother should submit to one, should be based on the interests of the child rather than on those of the prospective carers.

Divulging information when permission is given

The following recommendations, based on discussion at the seminar, were endorsed by the BAAF Medical Group Executive:

– that *the substitute parent or responsible residential worker* should not be left in ignorance. Wherever possible these children should be placed only with carers who have already had an opportunity to learn about and discuss the disease, both regarding day-to-day care and implications for the child's future

– that *the child's or the carer's general practitioner* should be informed, preferably by the agency's medical adviser

– that agencies should decide in each case whether others (for instance day carers or teachers) should be informed. This would depend mainly on the interests of the child and on the agreement of the birth parent, but attitudes currently prevailing in the community will also be relevant. Substitute parents carrying a burden of secrecy as well as responsibility for a potentially sick child require firm, regular and clearly identified support from both medical and social services. Single parents in particular may be helped by permission to share this information with another person – perhaps a close relative or another substitute parent.

The needs of the carers

Special needs

Carers of children at risk of being HIV positive are under additional stress. The prognosis for the child is uncertain and they also have to deal with unpredictable community attitudes if the child's circumstances are known. In addition, normal facilities for respite care, such as occasionally leaving the child with a relative or friend, are restricted. Some of the practical supports that should be available to carers are listed under *Support for placements* below.

Information

One of the major uncertainties in caring for an at-risk child lies in the fact that knowledge about HIV infection is developing and therefore information changing. The need for education programmes for carers is emphasised above, including a system for keeping them informed of relevant facts as these emerge.

Consultation

Because of the special stresses involved, carers of these children should have access to immediate social work support. This means that someone should be available for consultation out of office hours, whether through a specialist team or the emergency services. Both the social worker involved and the family's GP should also have ready access to specialist medical advice when necessary.

Financial supports

Families caring for at-risk children are likely to incur extra expenses, especially with symptomatic children. Extra allowances may well be justified.

Respite care

Anne Black of the Lothian Regional Social Work Department describes how her department set up a special unit staffed by nursery nurses for emergency and respite care of young at-risk children. Although hardly used, the existence of the unit gave confidence to the families caring for the children as well as to their social workers.

Responsibilities towards older children in care

This topic merits more consideration than we are able to give it here. We have stated above that carers have a special role in helping young people to understand the implications of HIV infection. Their task will be even more delicate in helping younger children who have been infected, either by parents before birth or by abusers in childhood, to come to terms with their situation as they grow up. These tasks will be impossible to perform unless carers and their social workers have earned the trust of these children and young people.

One group at the seminar encouraged agencies to look critically at their perceptions of children and young people in their care. How much involvement do they allow them in planning their own lives and are their views listened to, weighed up and taken into account when decisions are made? Alternatively, have they been allowed to take over the decision-making to such an extent that their insecurity is increased?

It could be that some residential establishments for young people in care will be at risk of the spread of HIV infection. This can be controlled only with the cooperation of the young people themselves and they will be more likely to comply if their cooperation as respected individuals has been sought also in other less dramatic areas of their lives.

Bereavement counselling

Dr Mok in Chapter 3 outlines the support that will be required by families caring for a dying child. Agencies need now to identify available resources for bereavement counselling especially relating to children.

Summary of Recommendations

Following the seminar, the Executive Committee of the BAAF Medical Group further considered the various issues raised. As a result it made the following recommendations and suggests that agencies use them as a basis for interdisciplinary discussions on the implications of HIV infection and disease.

Decision-making

Decisions relating to the placement of children at risk of any serious infectious disease should be made by a panel that would include a medical component, probably the agency's medical adviser, and such decisions should be made according to the circumstances pertaining in each individual case.

Education

Programmes should be drawn up for the education and training of all staff regarding the disease and its implications, including programmes designed for foster and adoptive parents, both already active and prospective.

Standards of hygiene
Strategies should be designed for acquiring and maintaining a high standard of general hygiene in the care of all children.

Keeping abreast of developments
A member of staff should be allocated special responsibility for keeping abreast of relevant developments in the field of HIV infection, in cooperation with colleagues in the Health Service.

Testing for HIV infection
Policies should be formed and recorded regarding which adults and children (if any) should be encouraged to submit to a test, including who should make this decision in individual cases and who should provide appropriate counselling.

Divulgence of information
Consideration should be given as to whether certain people should share full information about the child/parent's HIV status in every case (eg the carer, the GP).

Support for placements
The availability of various kinds of support should be considered, for example:
– round the clock availability of medical/social work consultation
– enhanced fostering allowances/adoption allowances
– respite care
– appropriate legal services
– an information service regarding the disease
– peer group support
– bereavement counselling

Responsibilities regarding older children in care
An atmosphere of mutual trust should be promoted between the children and the agency, which will include:
– the education and support of the carers

– the education of the children themselves and availability of follow-up through consultancy services
– the availability of medical services

Procedural guidelines
Guidelines for staff, carers and children should be drawn up, with facilities for updating them.

At the beginning of this chapter we referred to the opportunity available to workers in the UK to plan ahead on behalf of HIV infected children, an opportunity largely denied to our colleagues in the US. This opportunity not only offers breathing space but also presents a challenge, as indicated in the tasks set out above.

BAAF asks member agencies to seize the opportunity presented to meet this challenge.

A glossary of medical terms and organisations associated with HIV infection

AIDS (Acquired Immune Deficiency Syndrome)	An illness that impairs the body's ability to fight disease and which leaves the individual susceptible to some rare cancers and infections. Such infections are known as opportunistic infections
Antibodies	Any substance in the blood serum or other body fluids that destroys or neutralises bacteria, viruses or other harmful toxins that enter the body
Antigens	Any substance which, when introduced into the body, causes the production of a specific antibody. The HIV virus is such a substance
Antiviral	A type of substance that can destroy or weaken the pathogenic action of a virus. Antiviral drugs are being used experimentally against the AIDS virus
ARC (AIDS Related Complex)	A condition similar to AIDS that can exhibit many of the same symptoms, but does not yet meet the full conditions of AIDS and does not qualify for AIDS diagnosis. These symptoms may persist for many years but never develop into AIDS
Body fluids	Blood, saliva, semen, tears and vaginal fluids
British Paediatric Surveillance Unit (BPSU)	Set up by the BPA, CDSC (see below) and Department of Epidemiology, Institute of Child Health. It provides a national reporting scheme relating to cases of uncommon disease
Candidiasis	An infection caused by candida albicans, usually called 'thrush', which may occur in the mouth, vagina, lungs or intestines. Commonly occurs in immuno-suppressed individuals
Cardiomyopathy	Any disease of the heart muscles other than those caused by specific infections

Carers	People other than birth parents, giving day-to-day care to children
Cell-free plasma	Blood from which the cells have been removed
Centers for Disease Control, Atlanta, Georgia (CDC)	Centre holding responsibility for epidemiological surveillance in the US
Cyclosporine	A drug commonly used after organ transplant operations to reduce the possibility of foreign tissue being rejected by the body's immune system. Controversial experimental studies have been conducted in France using cyclosporine to treat persons with AIDS
CMV (cytomegalo-virus)	A herpes-related virus which attacks immuno-suppressed patients. May cause opportunistic infections in AIDS sufferers
Communicable Disease Surveillance Centre (CDSC)	Equivalent in the UK of the CDC
Contagious	Transmission of an infectious disease by direct body contact with an infected person
Cryptococcus	A yeast that causes a rare form of meningitis and pneumonia and occurs as an opportunistic infection in AIDS patients
Elisa test	A blood test which indicates whether someone has been exposed to a particular virus. The test does not detect disease but only the antibodies formed when there has been exposure to a virus. The test can be used to detect HIV antibody and is used to screen blood donors
Epidemiology	The study of factors which determine the occurrence of disease in a population
False negative	A negative blood test result in a patient who has been infected
False positive	A positive blood test result in a patient who has not been infected

Haemophilia	An inherited disease in which blood fails to clot. The administration of therapeutic blood products will control the bleeding. At the outbreak of the AIDS epidemic, infected men donated their infected blood as blood donors. This was transfused to haemophiliacs who have consequently contracted AIDS
High risk groups	Those groups of individuals that epidemiological evidence indicates are at the highest risk for contracting AIDS. These include: gay and bisexual men, intravenous drug users, haemophiliacs, prostitutes and sexual partners of people infected with HIV
HIV	Human Immuno-Deficiency Virus (see HTVL III)
HPA-23	A rare antiviral drug that has been studied in AIDS research for its ability to inhibit retroviral replication
HTVL-III (Human T-Cell Lymphotrophic Virus, Type Three)	Term first used by American scientist Dr Robert Gallo for the virus identified to be the cause of AIDS. HTLV-III may be written as 'LAV/HTLV-III', combining the American and French terminology. Virus has now been renamed HIV (Human Immuno-deficiency Virus)
Incubation period	The latent or silent state of an infectious disease intervening between the moment of infection and the appearance of symptoms. In AIDS this incubation period can be from two months to five years or longer
Infectious	Capable of being transmitted from person to person
Interferon	A naturally occurring substance which biologically modified the immune response. It has been used in AIDS treatment to modify the immune response and, specifically, in the treatment of the AIDS related skin cancer, Kaposi's Sarcoma
Intra-partum	During birth
Intra-uterine	Within the uterus

IV drug users (intravenous drug users)	A high-risk group for contracting AIDS. Associated with the sharing of needles and syringes for intravenous injection
KS (Kaposi's Sarcoma)	A normally rare form of skin cancer, now commonly identified as an opportunistic disease affecting persons with AIDS
LAV (lymphadenopathy – associated virus)	Term first used by French scientist Dr Luc Montagnier for the virus identified to be the cause of AIDS. LAV may be written as 'LAV/HTLV-III', combining the American and French terminology (see HTLV-III)
Leucocytes	Commonly known as white blood cells, they play a major role in fighting infectious disease. Lymphocytes are one subclass of leucocytes. The two types of white blood cells commonly associated with AIDS are the 'B' and 'T' lymphocytes
Lymphoid interstitial pneumonitis	A lung complaint frequently found in paediatric HIV disease
MMWR (*The Morbidity and Mortality Weekly Report*)	A weekly publication in the USA by the Centers for Disease Control that serves as a reference source for information on current trends in the nation's health. It is often cited for its statistics on the number of AIDS-related deaths and illnesses in the USA
Opportunistic infections	Infections caused by a variety of viruses, bacteria, fungi and protozoa that are either not ordinarily harmful or are easily controlled by a healthy immune system. The two most common opportunistic infections seen in AIDS are PCP and Kaposi's Sarcoma
PCP (Pneumocystis Carinii Pneumonia)	One of two opportunistic diseases first identified by the Centers for Disease Control in the formal definition of AIDS. It is caused by the protozoan parasite and is the most common cause of death for persons with the syndrome
Percutaneous	Through the skin
Perinatal	Around the time of birth
Pertussis	Whooping cough

Quadriparesis	Paralysis of all four limbs
Retrovirus	A type of virus unknown in humans until recently. HIV is a retrovirus and as such is believed to reproduce at a rapid rate
Seronegative	A blood screening test result indicating no presence of HIV antibodies in the blood stream
Seropositive	A blood screening test indicating presence of HIV antibodies in the bloodstream. This only indicates that a person has been exposed to the virus. It is not a test for AIDS. A seropositive person does *not* necessarily have AIDS and is not necessarily an AIDS patient
STD	Sexually transmitted diseases
Suramin	A rare anti-infectious drug that is being studied in AIDS research because it is believed to inhibit retroviral replication
T Cell	A type of white blood cell that is essential in the body's fight against infection
Thrush	See 'Candida'

We are grateful for the help of the Welsh AIDS Campaign in drawing up this Glossary.

Appendix 1 AIDS: what it means for young people

(Main content of leaflet produced by the Welsh AIDS Campaign PO Box 348, Cardiff CF1 4XL (tel. 0222 223443) described in Chapter 6.)

What is AIDS?

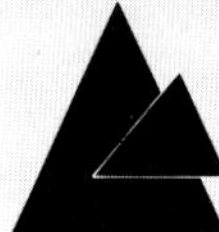

AIDS is – Acquired
Immune
Deficiency
Syndrome

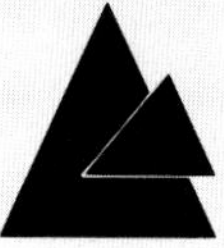

AIDS is – caused by a virus which destroys part of the body's immune system, so the body can't defend itself against illnesses people don't normally get.

These illnesses kill

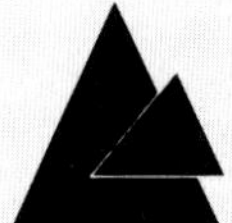

AIDS is – spreading rapidly.

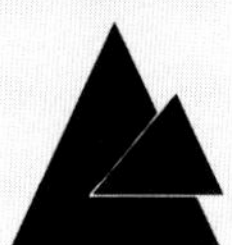

AIDS is – a disease for which there is **no** known cure.

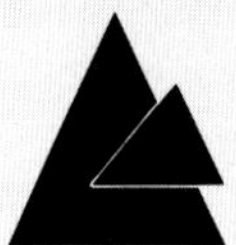

AIDS is – a disease which can be avoided if you are sensible.

YOU can avoid getting AIDS

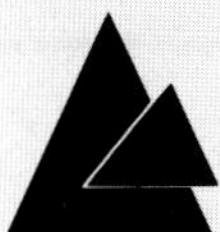

Don't sleep around with different partners.

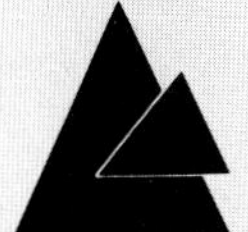

Always make sure, if you have sex, that you or your partner uses a sheath (condom, rubber, french letter, johnnie).

A sheath **may** break. You can make this less likely by using a proper lubricating jelly. **Don't** use vaseline – it dissolves rubber.

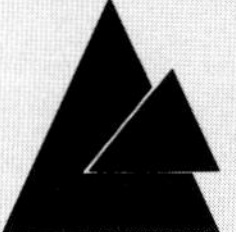

Don't use drugs. Don't share a needle or syringe.

Why take pointless chances? You don't have to catch AIDS.

BE SENSIBLE

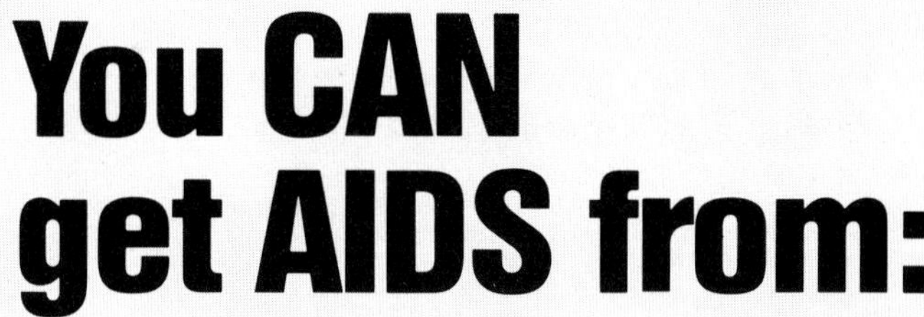

▶ having sex with someone who has the virus.

▶ getting infected blood into your bloodstream. Drug addicts who share needles and syringes are taking huge risks.

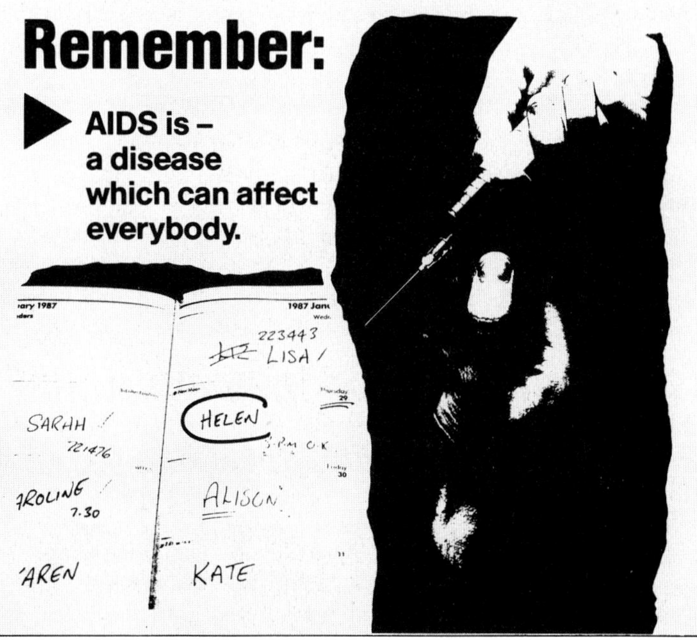

You CANNOT get AIDS from:

- casual contact – shaking hands, touching, hugging.
- giving blood, coughing or sneezing.
- toilet seats, swimming pools, glasses, cups, knives, forks.
- sharing books and pencils.
- kissing.

Ear piercing and tattooing must only be carried out with properly sterilised instruments **– don't do it yourself.**

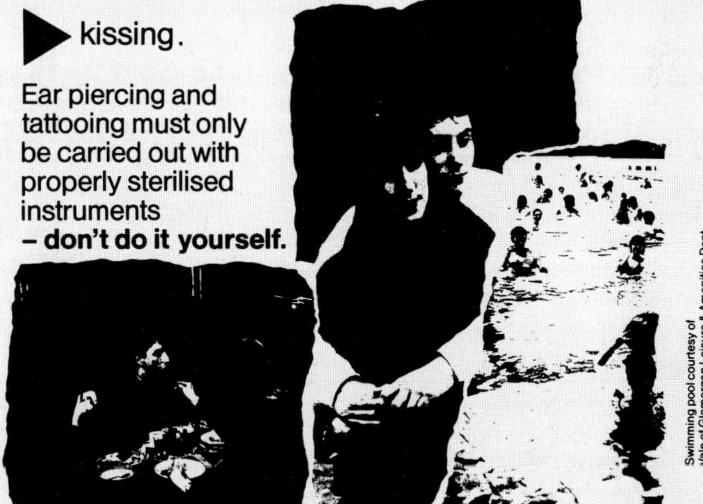

Swimming pool courtesy of Vale of Glamorgan Leisure & Amenities Dept.

Appendix II Focus, A Guide to AIDS Research

Focus, a guide to AIDS research is published monthly by the AIDS Health Project, Box 0884, San Francisco, CA 94143-0884, USA. This paper on counselling is taken from Volume 2, Number 5, April 1987. American spellings and terminology have been retained.

Whether to take the test: Counseling Guidelines

Peter Goldblum, PHd, MPH is the Education Development Specialist for the AIDS Health Project. *Neil Seymour, MA, MFCC*, is the Coordinator for the AIDS Antibody Counselling Program for the AIDS Health Project.

As the availability and use of the AIDS antibody test become more widespread, many more individuals are evaluating the benefits and risks of learning their antibody status. Some of these individuals will seek counsel from mental health professionals to help them decide whether to take the test. Clients already involved in counseling may wish to discuss these issues as part of their ongoing work. In addition, clients whose physicians have recommended the test for medical reasons may want to discuss their concerns about the possible negative psychological and social effects of taking the test. We outline here guidelines to help mental health practitioners in their work with clients concerned about taking the test and coping with the results.

Background and History

In early 1983 researchers identified the virus (now named the Human Immunodeficiency Virus, HIV) believed to cause AIDS. Shortly thereafter, private companies developed a sophisticated laboratory test called ELISA (enzyme-linked immunosorbent assay) to detect antibodies to the virus. The primary purpose of the test was to screen blood and blood products for HIV contamination. The test in and of itself is not a test for AIDS and the test result does not reveal whether a person will develop AIDS.

Infection by the AIDS virus causes a response by the body's immune system. Part of this response is the production of antibodies which recognize and attach to specific proteins on the virus, called antigens. Since the antibodies are tailor-made for particular antigens, tests can be designed to detect these specific antibodies. Tests for antibodies include the ELISA, the IFA (immunofluorescence assay), and the Western Blot. Each of these tests is based on the same principle, and each uses different methods to detect the same antibodies. Thus, the IFA or the Western Blot can be used as a way to support results obtained by the less-expensive ELISA.

The antibody tests are all very sensitive, which means that they detect almost all of the positive sera. They are also very specific, seldom indicating negative sera as positive. While testing procedures may vary, the required repeat testing of positive tests increases the accuracy of the test. False reactions do occur for reasons that are not completely understood. A false negative result may occur because an individual has not yet developed antibodies to the virus. Most people produce antibodies within two to eight weeks after exposure; some, however, will take up to six months.

Conversely, a false positive reaction may occur if the antibodies have developed in response to other similar proteins in the blood. Also, antibodies may have developed in reaction to another part of the test system, such as the cells in which the virus is grown. This would be called a non-specific reaction.

For individuals with little risk, the probability that a positive result is a 'false positive' is greater only because there seems little chance that such individuals would have been exposed to HIV. Especially in these cases, testing by another method or repeat testing in a few months should be encouraged. The recommended procedure for all positive results is to be tested by another method such as IFA or Western Blot. While false positive and false negative reactions may occur, accumulating evidence shows that the ELISA test is very accurate, especially for individuals at high risk.

Concerned that people at high risk might donate blood to learn their antibody status, public health officials developed an alternative test site program providing either anonymity or at least strict confidentiality to participants. Over time other purposes of the test have emerged. These include diagnostic and epidemiological applications as well as use in family planning settings to help clients make informed choices about pregnancy, parenthood, and birth control. Many see the test as an important preventive education tool for use in helping people understand their risk of contracting and transmitting the AIDS virus.

Ever since the antibody tests were developed, confusion and conflict about individual civil rights and public health interests have prevailed. Several public health officials and medical investigators wanted to use the test to help track and control the spread of the disease and to study the effects of infection. Advocates for people at high risk of HIV infection emphasized that many of these individuals are already socially stigmatized and that further use of the test might foster discrimination against those with positive results. Others, such as employers and insurance companies, showed an interest in the test for their own purposes.

Fears of discrimination have a realistic basis. Individuals in high-risk groups, regardless of their medical status, have lost jobs, have been denied housing and insurance, and have suffered from disruptions in relationships with families, partners, and friends. Homophobia, racism, and dislike or fear of drug addicts have been exacerbated by the hysteria and panic that have accompanied the AIDS epidemic. It is no wonder then that individuals in high-risk groups have been distrustful and suspicious in regard to the use of the antibody test. Given these facts, mental health professionals who counsel clients about the antibody test should provide information about possible consequences of taking the test and ways of managing the test information to prevent later difficulties.

Preparation for Counseling

To prepare for counseling, mental health professionals should first become familiar with the test, what it means and does not mean, its level of accuracy, and the potential benefits and risks of knowing one's antibody status. It is helpful to have ready access to community resources that can provide updated information relative to the test. Government-sponsored test sites have been established in several communities to offer information about the test and to provide anonymous testing free of charge. Clients can receive basic information at these sites and then return to their primary mental health counselors to review the information and weigh the personal benefits and risks prior to making a final decision.

Mental health professionals must examine their own bias toward the AIDS antibody test before they counsel clients about it. Counselors should understand fully the limits of the test and the real risks that the test can present. Clients must understand that the test alone will not indicate if they have AIDS or ARC, and that it will not predict who will develop these diseases.

In some cases antibody testing has resulted in a positive psychological and behavioral adaptation to the threat of AIDS. For those who prove to be antibody negative, knowledge of their tests results usually reduces unneeded anxiety, although some recipients may face problems with 'survivor guilt' and extra stress about remaining negative. Many individuals who receive a positive result have been motivated to take their health more seriously and to improve their health behaviors. Since research has shown that most people with AIDS antibodies have active virus in their bodies, a positive result strongly implies that an individual is able to pass the virus to another. Knowledge of a positive status has motivated many individuals to be more judicious in following safer sex guidelines and in no longer sharing IV needles. However, for many individuals troubling psychological reactions to test results frequently accompany the news of seropositivity. These responses range from mild to moderate anxiety to full-blown anxiety and depressive disorders. Although adequate pre-counseling can lessen the likelihood of these reactions, it is no guarantee that these will not happen.

Outline of Benefits and Risks

The benefits of antibody testing include:

1 to protect the blood supply by testing individuals who are considering donating blood;
2 to ensure that organ donations are safe from HIV contamination;

3 to help support a medical diagnosis in individuals who exhibit unexplained symptoms that their doctors think might be related to a HIV infection;
4 to help women at high risk decide whether to become pregnant or give birth;
5 to help women with a history of risk behavior decide whether to breastfeed an infant;
6 to reduce anxiety in individuals who are at low risk for HIV infection yet who have extremely high anxiety about it;
7 to motivate individuals who continue to practice high-risk behavior and who feel that a positive test result may help them reduce these behaviors;
8 to help researchers design experimental treatment protocols and to help potential subjects determine whether or not to participate in the drug trials;
9 to help scientists determine the extent of HIV infection in the population at large and, by following seropositive individuals, to understand the natural history of HIV infection.

The risks of antibody testing include:
1 severe psychological reactions, including anxiety, nightmares, sleep disturbance, depression, and suicidal behavior;
2 disrupted interpersonal relations, including potential for rage reactions and their extreme manifestations, such as homicidal behavior;
3 social ostracism and self-imposed social withdrawal;
4 relationship problems (blaming partners, sexual dysfunction, disrupted ability to make plans as a couple);
5 stigmatization and discrimination if a positive antibody status is made known to others outside of guarantees of confidentiality;
6 problems with employment or insurance;
7 preoccupations with bodily symptoms; and
8 a false sense of security and denial if the test proves negative (for example, believing one is immune to infection and thus continuing with risk behavior).

The Counseling Process

The process for helping clients decide whether to take the antibody test should be based on three important elements: (1) accurate information about the test, (2) a systematic decision-making process, and (3) an action plan that will maximize benefits and minimize risk.

Although the availability of information about the antibody test varies from one location to another, basic information and the location of the nearest test site should be available at any Public Health Department office. Some clinicians feel that clients should take responsibility for locating and obtaining information; others feel more comfortable providing information directly. In any case, clinicians should emphasize the importance of not proceeding with the test without proper background knowledge.

Clinicians should take responsibility for providing a structure for facilitating the decision-making process. This may be a process that has been used already with ongoing clients or one which is geared specifically for the immediate purpose. One process that has been used successfully is based on a 'benefit-risk analysis'. The client is asked to list the potential benefits that might be involved with taking the test. Subsequently, the client lists the potential risks. For the benefits list, the counselor encourages the client to consider each item and determine whether the benefit can be received by some means (other than the antibody test) that does not have concomitant risk. For example, if an individual is taking the test to lower the risk of contracting the disease through sexual contact, understanding that the same guidelines hold true for those who test positive as those who test negative may obviate the need to take the test.

If a greater overall benefit has been established to proceed with the test, a careful review of risks must be undertaken. In some cases perceived risks are in fact groundless, such as the fear that someone could obtain an individual's name from an anonymous test site. (A participant's anonymity is protected at these test sites; the individual's name is never recorded.) Other risks can be reduced somewhat by careful planning; for example, discussions by couples prior to testing about how they will cope with the test results.

After a careful examination of the benefits and risks, the final choice – an educated decision – is the client's own to make.

An Action Plan

If a client chooses to take the test, additional attention should focus on how to minimize risks once the results are known. Clients may begin to process their feelings and thoughts by imagining their reactions to receiving a positive result and developing strategies to cope with these reactions. This process may take several sessions before the client is psychologically prepared to take the test. Even this preparation is no guarantee that unexpected reactions may not overwhelm the client.

Appendix III General reading list

Books

Anderson G R *Children and AIDS: the challenge for child welfare* Child Welfare League of America, 1986.

Citizens' Committee for Children of New York, Inc *The invisible emergency: children and AIDS in New York* Citizens' Committee for Children of New York, 1987.

Daniels V G *AIDS: the Acquired Immune Deficiency Syndrome* MTP Press, 1985.

Daniels V G *AIDS: questions and answers* Cambridge Medical Books, 1986.

Hawkes N *AIDS – illustrated booklet aimed at young people* Franklin Watts.

Jones P (ed) *Proceedings of the AIDS conference 1986 (sponsored by the DHSS and the Haemophilia Society)* Intercept Ltd, 1986.

Pinching A J (ed) *AIDS and HIV infection (clinics in immunology and allergy vol. 6: 3)* W B Saunders, 1986.

Weber J and Ferriman A *Aids concerns you: what every man and every woman should know about AIDS* Pagoda Books, 1986.

Newsletters

AIDS Bulletin issued by the Scottish Education Department and Social Work Service Group – an exchange of information and views on AIDS related matters. Enquiries to Rob Walker, SWSG, Scottish Education Department, 43 Jeffrey Street, Edinburgh, EH1 1DN (tel: 031 244 5435).

AIDS and Retrovirus Update Monthly annotated bibliography *AIDS Newsletter* Summarises recent major news items from the UK and abroad and latest clinical and scientific developments, statistics etc, for health care workers. Both from: Bureau of Hygiene and Tropical Medicine, Keppel Street, London WC1E 7HT (tel: 01 636 8636 ext 275).

Focus – a guide to AIDS research issued monthly by the AIDS Health Project. FOCUS: A guide to AIDS Research, Box 0884, San Francisco, CA 94143-0884, USA.

APPENDIX IV Organisations concerned with AIDS relating to children and young people

AIDS Information Service (DHSS): telephone advice service (0800 535535).

The Health Education Council, 78 New Oxford Street, London WC1A 1AH, have a comprehensive list of films, videos, tapes, slides and leaflets (tel: 01 631 0930).

The Voluntary Council for Handicapped Children, 8 Wakley Street, London EC1V 7QE (01 278 9441) is preparing lists of information to be available by Christmas 1987.

The National Foster Care Association, Francis House, Francis Street, London SW1 (01 828 6266) publish a leaflet in their Signposts series called *AIDS and HIV – information for foster parents.*

The Institute of Child Health, 30 Guildford Street, London WC1 (01 242 9789).

The Haemophilia Society, 123 Westminster Bridge Road, London SE1 7HR (01 928 2020).

The Terrence Higgins Trust, BM AIDS, London WC1N 3XX (01 833 2971).